Recent Advances in Endourology, 6

H. Kumon, M. Murai, S. Baba (Eds.)

Endourooncology

New Horizons in Endourology

Recent Advances in Endourology, 6

H. Kumon, M. Murai, S. Baba (Eds.)

Endourooncology
New Horizons in Endourology

With 53 Figures

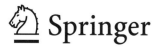 Springer

Hiromi Kumon, M.D., Ph.D.
Professor and Chairman, Department of Urology
Okayama University Graduate School of Medicine and Dentistry
2-5-1 Shikata, Okayama 700-8558, Japan

Masaru Murai, M.D., Ph.D.
Professor and Chairman, Department of Urology
Keio University School of Medicine
35 Shinanomachi, Shinjuku-ku, Tokyo 160-8586, Japan

Shiro Baba, M.D., Ph.D.
Professor and Chairman, Department of Urology
Kitasato University School of Medicine
1-15-1 Kitasato, Sagamihara, Kanagawa 228-8555, Japan

ISBN 4-431-21389-9 Springer-Verlag Tokyo Berlin Heidelberg New York

Library of Congress Control Number: 2004113089

Printed on acid-free paper

Springer is a part of Springer Science+Business Media
springeronline.com

Typesetting: SNP Best-set Typesetter Ltd., Hong Kong
Printing and binding: Shinano Inc., Japan
SPIN: 10997055 series number 4130

Preface

The trend in all surgical disciplines has been toward nonoperative or minimally invasive treatment. Endourology, which began with the development of cystoscopy, now encompasses all minimally invasive techniques including urologic laparoscopy, creating new horizons in endourology. Endourooncology, the merging of endourology and oncology, is one of the most challenging and rapidly evolving areas in urology practice and will revolutionize our approach to urologic malignancies with continuing refinements in technique.

Recent Advances in Endourology, volume 6, one of a series of publications organized by the Japanese Society of Endourology and ESWL, focuses on endourooncology and related topics. For the treatment of urologic malignancies, advanced and sophisticated reconstructive procedures increasingly have been performed purely laparoscopically. In the near future, standardized procedures will be conducted by robotic systems with advanced surgical eyes and hands. A more important role of robotic systems will be to open new vistas for telementoring and telerobotic cancer surgery, providing a novel educational system in order to overcome the steep learning curve faced by inexperienced surgeons. In addition, a variety of energy-based, targeted technologies, including radiofrequency ablation, high-intensity focused ultrasound (HIFU), and cryoablation are being investigated intensively for the treatment of localized urologic cancers. These image-guided targeted therapies will become preferred options as early detection methods for localized cancers develop, as in the case of transperineal brachytherapy for prostate cancer. Similarly, image-guided in situ gene therapy will have a great impact on future endourooncology.

We editors are most grateful to the authors for contributing excellent, informative review articles. We believe that these thirteen articles will enable the reader to envision future horizons in endourooncology. In the future, we will be able to offer each patient the most beneficial, tailor-made procedure that will provide lower morbidity, less pain, shorter hospital stay, and excellent cosmesis as well as a favorable long-term oncological and functional outcome.

Hiromi Kumon, M.D., Ph.D.
Chief Editor

Contents

Contributors

Merging of Endourology and Oncology: Endourooncology

Assaad El-Hakim, Benjamin R. Lee, and Arthur D. Smith

Summary. There is a growing need to bring together endourological approaches and sound oncological principles to achieve minimally invasive cancer control in urologic malignancies. Reduced treatment morbidity and quality-of-life issues are becoming more valued by both patients and physicians. In this chapter, we present an overview of the most recent advances in endoscopic, laparoscopic, and energy-based ablation techniques for the treatment of upper-tract transitional-cell carcinoma, renal-cell carcinoma, prostate cancer, adrenal tumors, and germ-cell testicular tumors. The merge between endourology and urologic oncology will undeniably revolutionize our approach to urologic malignancies.

Keywords. Renal cell carcinoma, Transitional cell carcinoma, Prostate cancer, Testicular cancer, Laparoscopy

Introduction

Endourologists have always strived to decrease the morbidity of surgical procedures and improve patients' quality of life. Endourology, initially defined as "the closed and controlled manipulation within the urinary tract," has favorably encompassed all minimally invasive techniques, including laparoscopy, for the betterment of patients' care. The field of urologic oncology is not an exception to this leading force of least invasiveness. Based on the principles of the oldest oncologic endoscopic surgery, namely, transurethral resection of bladder tumors, the endoscopic approach to superficial upper-tract transitional cell carcinoma has evolved for the past two decades. More recently, laparoscopic approaches to all urologic cancers have been developed and validated, and have achieved cancer control comparable to that with traditional open surgeries. Laparoscopic radical nephrectomy has replaced open radical nephrectomy for low-stage

Department of Urology, Long Island Jewish Medical Center, 270-05 76th Avenue, New Hyde Park, NY 11040-1496, USA

(T1–T2) renal neoplasia in many institutions around the world. Other energy-based technologies, including cryosurgery, radiofrequency ablation, and high-intensity focused ultrasound (HIFU), are being investigated intensively for the treatment of localized renal and prostate cancers. Hence, the field of endouro-oncology has become a reality. In this chapter we give a general overview of recent developments in minimally invasive urologic oncology.

Upper-Tract Transitional Cell Carcinoma

Endoscopic Treatment

The traditional treatment of upper-tract transitional cell carcinoma (TCC) has been nephroureterectomy with bladder cuff excision. Endoscopic (percutaneous or ureteroscopic) treatment of upper-tract TCC emerged initially from the need for renal preservation in a subset of patients with anatomical or functional solitary kidneys. Lessons learned from this early experience paved the way for elective endoscopic treatment of superficial low-risk upper-tract TCC in patients with normal contralateral renal units [1, 2]. Strict indications include solitary, small (less than 2 cm), low-grade, completely visible, and resectable lesions. In the Mayo Clinic series, 21 patients meeting these inclusion criteria underwent endourologic management of upper-tract TCC, resulting in an overall renal salvage rate of 81%. The 5-year disease-specific survival was 100%; however, the overall 5-year survival curve was lower than expected (66% vs 78%) for a similar disease-free age group in the United States [2].

Contraindications to endourologic treatment of upper-tract TCC include high-grade (grade 3 or 4) lesions and tumors that appear to be invasive on radiographic imaging or direct endoscopic inspection. If a tumor is found to be unresectable on either anatomic or technical grounds, laparoscopic nephroureterectomy should follow. Recurrence at a higher grade of a previously resected tumor or a tumor that recurs rapidly after resection and bacille Calmette-Guérin (BCG) instillation portends aggressive disease, and further attempts at conservative therapy are ill-advised.

The percutaneous approach provides improved visibility and the ability to use larger instruments. On the other hand, the ureteroscopic approach is less invasive. It has been our practice to initially proceed with ureteroscopy. If the tumor is not completely resectable ureteroscopically, a percutaneous resection is undertaken under the same anesthesia.

The preoperative metastatic work-up includes, at a minimum, a computerized tomographic (CT) scan of the abdomen and pelvis and chest radiography.

Patients with grade 1 disease have an excellent prognosis, whereas the prognosis of those with grade 3 disease is guarded. Grade 1 disease has a reported recurrence rate of 16% on average (range, 5% to 33%) [3–6]. However, despite recurrences, death from low-grade urothelial carcinoma is rare. The prognosis of grade 2 disease is also good. The average recurrence rate is 22% (range, 6% to

33%) [3–7]. However, no matter how grade 3 urothelial carcinoma of the upper urinary tract is managed, the prognosis is poor. We recently updated our series of endoscopically treated upper-tract TCC. Ninety patients with upper-tract TCC were treated with primary endoscopic intent (ureteroscopic and/or percutaneous approach) at our institution between April 1985 and May 2003. Seventy-two patients (75 renal units) were closely followed thereafter, and 18 patients underwent definitive surgical extirpative treatment shortly after initial endoscopic resection. According to multivariate analysis, tumor grade and focality were predictive of survival ($p < 0.05$). Patient age, gender, tumor stage, tumor side, and year of resection were not predictive of survival (unpublished data). In the authors' opinion, endoscopic resection should not be offered for high-grade multifocal upper-tract TCC, except as an alternative in elderly patients with a solitary kidney who would fare quite poorly on hemodialysis. In fact, the 5-year survival rate of patients with end-stage renal failure in the age group from 75 to 84 years is only 10% [60].

A rigorous, lifelong follow-up regimen should be tailored to the recurrence pattern of upper-tract tumors. Although long-term (over 5 years) recurrences have been reported, most recurrences occur in the first 3 years following initial therapy [8]. These patients should undergo routine bladder surveillance as well. Ureteroscopy is the best modality to survey the ipsilateral upper tract [9]. The authors recommend that ureteroscopy be performed every 6 months, that the contralateral kidney be imaged at least annually with either retrograde or excretory pyelography, and that an abdominal CT scan be performed yearly.

The indications for adjuvant therapy (BCG, mitomycin C) in upper-tract urothelial cancer have evolved over the years. Grade 2 tumors, multifocal disease, T1 tumors, carcinoma in situ, and bilateral disease used to constitute the main indications for adjuvant *percutaneous* BCG at the authors' institution. In our recent update of the LIJ series, we identified 44 patients who received adjuvant BCG after endoscopic resection of upper-tract TCC and 29 who did not (controls). In this retrospective cohort, BCG increased overall survival of patients with low-grade tumors, unifocal tumors, and elective surgical indications. Furthermore, the recurrence rate was decreased in unifocal tumors receiving BCG compared with controls ($P < 0.05$) [61]. In light of these findings, the indications for adjuvant BCG need to be reconsidered, and a prospective multicenter trial is warranted.

In conclusion, endourologic techniques are ideal for managing noninvasive, resectable tumors that are well or moderately differentiated. These modalities are particularly suited to patients with renal compromise, as well as to patients with normally functioning kidneys and favorable tumor characteristics.

Laparoscopic Nephroureterectomy

Although laparoscopic radical nephrectomy has been widely accepted and adopted as a treatment option for renal cell carcinoma (RCC), the use of laparoscopic nephroureterectomy (LNU) for upper-tract TCC has lagged because of the lower incidence of the disease and management of the distal ureter and bladder cuff. LNU can be performed through a transperitoneal or retroperitoneal approach. There are several alternatives for dealing with the distal ureter and ensuring a bladder cuff [10]. The Pluck technique is a transvesical ureteral dissection whereby the ureteral orifice and intramural ureter are resected transurethrally using a Collins knife. In order to prevent tumor spillage from the upper tract, we recommend performing the laparoscopic nephrectomy first and applying a clip on the distal ureter early during dissection. Alternatively, an Endoloop (Ethicon Endosurgery, Cincinnati, OH, USA) can be used transvesically to occlude the distal ureter. A novel approach without the need for intraoperative patient repositioning (in lithotomy) has been recently reported [11]. A rigid offset nephroscope is introduced through a 10-mm working port into the bladder, and an incision is made around the ureteral orifice using the Collins knife, through the working channel of the nephroscope. Open bladder cuff resection, laparoscopic stapled bladder cuff, and ureteral intussusception [12] are all described alternatives. The specimen should be removed intact without morcellation through the hand port incision if hand-assisted LNU is performed, or through a lower midline or Pfannenstiel incision.

Four recent clinical series compared LNU with open nephroureterectomy (ONU) [13–16]. There were a total of 108 LNU procedures and 105 ONU procedures in these four series. The mean follow-up period was 11.1 to 35 months for LNU and 14 to 46 months for ONU. All four reports demonstrated a shorter hospital stay for LNU, by a mean of 1 to 6 days. The mean blood loss decreased on average from 440–696 ml for ONU to 199–288 ml for LNU. None of the LNU patients had their specimens morcellated. There were two extravesical local recurrences with LNU and three with ONU, as well as five distant metastatic diseases with LNU and seven with ONU. There were 8 disease-related deaths with LNU and 14 with ONU. There were no reported port site recurrences in these four series, despite earlier reports of tumor seeding into the port sites [17, 18].

LNU has obvious benefits over ONU, including decreased pulmonary complications, decreased postoperative discomfort, shorter hospital stay, and shorter convalescence. At medium-term follow-up of patients with upper tract TCC, the disease-free survival rate of those treated with LNU seems to be similar to that of patients treated with ONU. Although concerns over port site and intraperitoneal seeding have been voiced, these problems have not been reported in recent series. The overall disease-specific survival is comparable to that for ONU. However, long-term results are required.

Renal-Cell Carcinoma

The concept of elective nephron-sparing surgery has become well established in the past decade. Currently, 60% of all renal tumors are detected incidentally and are often small (4 cm or less), with up to 22% of these tumors not being malignant [19, 20]. Among patients with small renal tumors (4 cm or less), the 5- and

10-year survival rates are comparable for patients undergoing partial nephrectomy and those undergoing radical nephrectomy. Disease-specific survival following nephron-sparing surgery for small tumors is in excess of 90% [21]. In addition, preservation of nephrons is protective against hyperfiltration injury. A negative parenchymal margin is the primary oncologic goal, regardless of the thickness of that margin.

Until recently, the only available nephron-sparing option was open partial nephrectomy. However, within the past 5 years, various minimally invasive alternatives have been the subject of intense basic and clinical investigation. Based on established oncologic principles, all minimally invasive nephron-sparing procedures must aim to excise or effectively ablate renal tumors similar to what would have been excised during open partial nephrectomy. Although exciting, these new developments should be tested in well-designed preclinical and clinical trials. Long-term follow-up data are of extreme importance before widespread application.

Laparoscopic Partial Nephrectomy

Laparoscopic partial nephrectomy (LPN) has not been widely adopted, mainly because of the technical difficulty in achieving adequate parenchymal hemostasis and renal hypothermia.

Nephron-sparing surgery provides cancer control comparable to radical nephrectomy in select patients with a small (less than 4 cm), localized renal-cell carcinoma [22]. LPN was initially reserved for select patients with small, peripheral, and exophytic tumors [23–26]. With increased experience, the indications have been expanded to include patients with more complex tumors. Absolute contraindications for LPN include renal vein thrombus, and central tumors.

Successful LPN requires strict patient selection and proficiency in intracorporeal suturing. Open partial nephrectomy principles should be duplicated. Intraoperatively, a flexible laparoscopic ultrasound probe can be used to precisely delineate the tumor. The transperitoneal approach is chosen for anterior and lateral tumors, whereas the retroperitoneal approach is preferred for posterior tumors. A ureteral catheter is inserted cystoscopically in patients who require retrograde pyelography. The operative steps include renal hilum preparation for subsequent cross-clamping, followed by mobilization of the kidney and exposure of the tumor. Transperitoneally, a laparoscopic Satinsky clamp is used to occlude the renal hilum en bloc, or laparoscopic bulldog clamps are applied on the renal artery and/or vein separately. The tumor is excised and entrapped within a laparoscopic bag. Retrograde injection of dilute indigo carmine or methylene blue is used to identify any pelvicalyceal entry, which is laparoscopically sutured in a watertight fashion. Parenchymal hemostatic sutures are placed over Surgicel bolsters. A drain is placed, particularly if pelvicalyceal repair was performed.

Various techniques of parenchymal hemostasis have been reported. Cauterization of the cut surface with an argon beam laser and application of fibrin glue have been explored. For larger vessels, however, the most effective method remains the application of hemostatic parenchymal sutures. Renal parenchymal tourniquets and cable tie devices have been tested in the porcine kidney but are clinically unreliable in the human kidney. Other hemostatic aids include prior microwave thermotherapy [27] or radiofrequency coagulation [28] of the tumor followed by laparoscopic partial nephrectomy. Bioadhesives may become an effective method for obtaining renal parenchymal hemostasis in the future.

Gill et al. reported on the initial 50 patients who underwent LPN without renal hypothermia [29]. The warm ischemia time was 23 min, the mean operative time was 3 h, and the mean hospital stay was 2.2 days. On pathologic examination, renal-cell carcinoma was confirmed in 68% of the patients, all with a negative surgical margin. The intraoperative complication rate was 5%, including parenchymal hemorrhage, a ureteral injury, and a bowel abrasion, but none was converted. There were 9% postoperative and 15% late complications. Janetschek et al. recently reported on 15 patients treated with LPN. Cold ischemia was achieved by continuous perfusion of Ringer's lactate at 4°C through the clamped renal artery. The mean operative time was 185 min, the mean ischemia time was 40 min, and the mean estimated blood loss was 160 ml. Pathologic examination revealed RCC in 13 patients and angiomyolipoma in 2. The resection margins were negative in 14 patients. There were no significant postoperative complications [30].

Energy-Based Ablation Techniques

Cryoablation and radiofrequency ablation (RFA) are the two most studied minimally invasive alternatives to partial nephrectomy. They can be performed using open, laparoscopic or percutaneous approach. Cryoablation of renal tumors has the longest follow-up among energy based ablation techniques. Studies on animals have shown that tissue destruction is complete, and may be reliably reproduced [31, 32]. Long-term results from clinical trials are soon going to be available. Cryotherapy and RFA both involve a direct cellular injury and an indirect effect from microvascular impairment [33]. Ultrasound can be used to verify extension of the iceball during cryosurgery; however, currently there are no direct means to monitor RFA treatment intraoperatively.

Rukstalis et al. reported on 29 patients with localized renal tumors treated with cryoablation using an open approach [34]. The median preoperative lesion size was 2.2 cm. At a median follow-up of 16 months all patients except one, who had a biopsy-proven local recurrence, demonstrated radiographic regression to only a residual scar or a small nonenhancing cyst. Using the laparoscopic cryoablation approach, Gill et al. [35] treated 32 patients with a mean tumor size of 2.3 cm. Twenty-three patients have undergone a 3 to 6-month follow-up CT-guided biopsy, which was negative in all cases. No evidence of local recurrence was found during a mean follow-up of 16.2 months. Shingleton et al. reported on 65 patients with percutaneous cryotherapy. At an average follow-up of 18 months all 60 surviving patients had no radiographic evidence of disease, although nine out of 65 (14%) required repeat treatment [36]. The intermediate results look promising, and long-term data will soon be available to assess the durability of renal cryotherapy. (Refer to chapter 5–2, this volume, for further details on cryoablation of RCC).

RFA has recently entered phase II clinical trials for the treatment of small renal tumors. Four recent clinical studies using percutaneous RF reported favorable results with post-procedure CT or MRI enhancement as the primary measure of treatment failure [37–40]. Unfortunately, the absence of contrast enhancement is not an accurate predictor of tumor viability. However, there is as of yet no other reliable postoperative imaging to identify failures. When histology is used as a measure of outcome, several studies have shown incomplete tumor ablation [41–43]. Both hematoxylin and eosin stain (H&E) and nicotinamide adenine dinucleotide (NADH) diaphorase staining should be part of the histological assessment of RF ablated tumors because there are 'viable-appearing' cells on H&E in *acutely* ablated lesions [44].

Complete tumor cell death has not been consistently achieved with RF ablation of RCC. Based on findings of viable tumor cells only at the periphery of treated tumors, it seems reasonable to believe that better intraoperative monitoring would decrease or eliminate positive margins. Until long-term efficacy is well documented, RF treatment should be limited to small (<3 cm) and exophytic renal tumors in the setting of clinical trials. (Refer to chapter 5–1, this volume, for further details on RFA of renal tumors).

Prostate Cancer

Quality of life is a major consideration in the treatment of localized prostate cancer. The issue arises of striking a balance between treating asymptomatic patients and introducing side effects versus deferring treatment until patients become symptomatic, by which time cure may not be possible. The current treatments for early disease have acute and delayed morbidities that affect negatively the quality of life. There would therefore appear to be a need for new treatment options particularly in view of the high incidence of early disease.

Laparoscopic Radical Prostatectomy

In the late 1990s, Guilloneau et al. described a technique for laparoscopic radical prostatectomy (LRP), an approach that has the potential to offer lower morbidity than open procedures [45]. They have recently reported on 1,000 consecutive patients with clinically localized prostate cancer who underwent LRP. Clinical stage was T1a in 6 patients (0.6%), T1b in 3 (0.3%), T1c in 660 (66.5%), T2a in 304 (30.4%) and T2b in 27 (2.7%). Mean preoperative prostate specific antigen (PSA) was 10 +/−6.1 ng/ml. Positive surgical margin rate was 6.9%, 18.6%, 30% and 34% for pathological stages pT2a, pT2b, pT3a and pT3b, respectively. The overall actuarial biochemical progression-free survival rate was 90.5%

at 3 years. Preservation of the neurovascular bundles did not affect the status of surgical margins or disease progression [46]. Accordingly, LRP is at least equivalent to published series of open radical prostatectomy in terms of local disease control and biochemical progression free survival. Other approaches to LRP have also been described with favorable oncologic results and low morbidity rates [47, 48].

Laparoscopic radical prostatectomy is feasible and reduces perioperative blood loss, but has a steep learning curve. Continence and potency rates compare to open series. However, controversy remains whether LRP offers significant advantages in postoperative analgesic requirements, hospital stay and recovery period. Prospective randomized trials comparing LRP and open retropubic prostatectomy are underway, and results should clarify theses issues.

Energy-Based Treatment Alternatives

Cryosurgery and HIFU are some of the minimally invasive alternatives for localized prostate cancer. These modalities offer several advantages over radical surgery. They have low general surgical morbidity, can be performed on an outpatient basis, and blood transfusions are not needed. The results of a retrospective multicenter analysis of cryosurgery for have been published [49]. The 5-year biochemical-free survival rate was 76% for low-risk patients, which was comparable to the results for similar patients undergoing brachytherapy or conformal radiation at the same institutions. Nerve-sparing cryosurgery has recently been described and may increase the popularity of cryosurgery. (See chapter 6–3, this volume, for more details).

The short-term results of a large phase II/III European prospective multicenter trial of HIFU were recently published. 402 patients with localized prostate cancer unfit for radical prostatectomy were treated. The mean serum PSA concentration was 10.9 ng/ml. The Gleason scores were 2 to 4 in 13.2% of the patients, 5 to 7 in 77.5%, and 8 to 10 in 9.3%. Patients received a mean of 1.4 HIFU sessions. At a mean follow-up of 407 days 87.2% of clinical stage T1–2 patients achieved a negative biopsy postoperatively [50]. These new minimally invasive techniques are still investigational at present and before their role in localized prostate cancer can be defined it will be necessary to conduct larger studies with longer follow-up as well as comparative studies against traditional therapeutic options. Their role as salvage therapy also warrants investigation. (See chapter 6–2 for more details).

Adrenal Cortical Carcinoma

Laparoscopic Adrenalectomy

Laparoscopic adrenalectomy has replaced open surgery for the treatment of most surgical adrenal pathologies. Pheochromocytomas once considered a contraindication for laparoscopic surgery can now be excised safely and effectively [51].

Primary adrenal carcinoma is a rare tumor occurring in children and adults, and has a poor prognosis despite aggressive multimodality treatment approach [52]. Most malignancies of the adrenal are metastases from other primaries. Melanoma, renal cell carcinoma and adenocarcinoma of the lung, stomach, esophagus and liver metastasize to the adrenal in decreasing order of frequency [53]. Adrenal metastases from any primary malignancy were rarely diagnosed during life. With the increased use of imaging modalities for cancer staging, a higher number of adrenal metastases are being diagnosed. They usually are multiple and bilateral [53]. However if the metastasis is solitary, whether synchronous or metachronous with the primary neoplasm, surgical excision confers a survival benefit with a 5 year survival rate approaching 45% for metastatic non-small cell lung cancer, and 62% disease free survival at 26-month follow-up for metastatic renal cell carcinoma [54]. Prerequisite to adrenalectomy for metastasis is adequate control of the primary, absence of other non-resectable metastases and a patient with good performance status. Preoperative fine needle aspiration (FNA) of the tumor can be helpful in the differential diagnosis. Laparoscopic adrenalectomy for an isolated metastasis is safe effective and efficient. Our technique of laparoscopic adrenalectomy has been previously described [51].

Laparoscopic adrenalectomy for primary adrenal carcinoma is still controversial for the following reasons: the large size of the tumor (90% of adrenal carcinomas are >6 cm) [55], local infiltration, adrenal vein thrombus, and risk of spillage and subsequent recurrence. Size and recurrence do not seem to be the limiting factors and several cases of laparoscopic adrenalectomy for tumors >6 cm have been reported with acceptable operative time and low conversion rate and recurrence [51]. However most experienced surgeons agree that invasive tumors with surrounding tissue infiltrationor adrenal vein thrombus are formal contraindications to laparoscopic adrenalectomy.

Testicular Cancer

Laparoscopic Retroperitoneal Lymph Node Dissection

In the United States, retroperitoneal lymph node dissection (RPLND) is the main diagnostic and therapeutic option for stage I, non-seminomatous germ-cell testicular tumors (NSGCTT). In the early 1990s, the laparoscopic approach to RPLND was introduced as an alternative to open surgery in order to reduce the morbidity of open RPLND, which is too high for a diagnostic procedure. Janetschek et al. reported on the first large series of laparoscopic RPLND with significant follow-up demonstrating similar cancer control in patients with clinical stage I testis cancer compared to traditional open surgery. Seventy-three patients underwent a modified unilateral template dissection. Operative time ranged from 150 to 630 min (mean 297), with a significant drop after the initial 15 cases. The conversion rate was 2.7%. In the last 44 patients there was no major postoperative complication. The mean hospital stay was 3.3 days. Ejaculation was preserved in all patients. Lymph nodes were positive in 19 cases (26% pathologic stage II). There was one contralateral retroperitoneal recurrence at a mean follow-up of 43.3 months in a patient with initial pathologic stage I [56]. The Johns Hopkins' group recently reported their long-term data of laparoscopic RPLND in 29 patients with high risk clinical stage I, NSGCTT. A modified template dissection was performed. Lymph nodes were negative in 17 of 29 patients. Of these 17 patients, 15 had no recurrence and were free of disease with 5.8 years of follow-up. Two patients had recurrence, one in the chest, and one biochemical, and both were free of disease after chemotherapy. Notably, ten out of twelve lymph node positive patients underwent adjuvant chemotherapy and were free of disease with 6.3 years of follow-up. One patient had a biochemical recurrence and was salvaged with chemotherapy. The only long-term complication was retrograde ejaculation in 1 patient [57], however there was a high major complication rate of 14%.

Although challenging, laparoscopic RPLND is also feasible after chemotherapy for clinical stage IIA or higher. Palese et al. reported on 7 such patients. The mean tumor diameter was 3.07 cm before chemotherapy and 1.91 cm after chemotherapy. A modified laparoscopic left (n = 3), right (n = 3), and bilateral (n = 1) template was used. Post chemotherapy laparoscopic RPLND was successfully completed in 5 (71.4%) patients. The overall complication rate was 57.1%), with a major complication incidence of 42.8% [58]. Janetschek et al. performed post chemotherapy laparoscopic RPLND in 24 patients. Mean tumor diameter was 2.4 cm. before and 1.1 cm. after chemotherapy. There were no conversions to open surgery. Operative time was 150 to 300 min (mean 240). Blood loss was minimal and no blood transfusions were required. The only postoperative complications were chylous ascites (5 patients) which resolved with conservative management and a small asymptomatic lymphocele. Histological examination revealed necrosis in 71%, mature teratoma in 25% and active tumor in 4% of patients. Antegrade ejaculation was preserved in all patients. Mean postoperative hospital stay was 4 days, return to normal activities between 1 and 3 weeks, and time to complete recovery between 5 and 10 weeks. All patients were well without evidence of disease at a mean follow-up of 24.4 months [59].

Although feasible, laparoscopic RPLND should be viewed as only diagnostic, and considered investigational at the present time. The long and steep learning curve remains the biggest obstacle to laparoscopic RPLND.

It is difficult to draw definite conclusions on the therapeutic effect of primary laparoscopic RPLND because most patients with viable disease received adjuvant chemotherapy.

Conclusion

Minimally invasive approaches should be incorporated in the diagnosis and treatment of urologic malignancies. Unfortunately most centers specializing in the treatment of these diseases are not trained in laparoscopic surgery and vice versa. There is an urgent need to reconcile both urologic oncology and endourology. Today's urooncologist must become an endooncologist.

References

1. Chen GL, Bagley DH (2000) Ureteroscopic management of upper tract transitional cell carcinoma in patients with normal contralateral kidneys. J Urol 164:1173–1176
2. Elliott DS, Segura JW, Lightner D, Patterson DE, Blute ML (2001) Is nephroureterectomy necessary in all cases of upper tract transitional cell carcinoma? Long-term results of conservative endourologic management of upper tract transitional cell carcinoma in individuals with a normal contralateral kidney. Urology 58:174–178
3. Jarrett TW, Sweetser PM, Weiss GH, Smith AD (1995) Percutaneous management of transitional cell carcinoma of the renal collecting system: 9-year experience. J Urol 154:1629–1635
4. Clark PE, Streem SB, Geisinger MA (1999) 13-year experience with percutaneous management of upper tract transitional cell carcinoma. J Urol 161:772–776
5. Patel A, Soonawalla P, Shepherd SF, Dearnaley DP, Kellett MJ, Woodhouse CRJ (1996) Long-term outcome after percutaneous treatment of transitional cell carcinoma of the renal pelvis. J Urol 155:868–874
6. Lee BR, Jabbour ME, Marshall FF, Smith AD, Jarrett TW (1999) 13-year survival comparison of percutaneous and open nephroureterectomy approaches for management of transitional cell carcinoma of renal collecting system: Equivalent outcomes. J Endourol 13:289–294
7. Jabbour ME, Desgrandchamps F, Cazin S, Teillac P, Le Duc A, Smith AD (2000) Percutaneous management of grade II upper urinary tract transitional cell carcinoma: the long-term outcome. J Urol 163:1105–1107
8. Mills IW, Laniado ME, Patel A (2001) The role of endoscopy in the management of patients with upper urinary tract transitional cell carcinoma. BJU Int 87:150–162
9. Chen GL, El-Gabry EA, Bagley DH (2000) Surveillance of upper urinary tract transitional cell carcinoma: the role of ureteroscopy, retrograde pyelography, cytology, and urinalysis. J Urol 164:1173–1176
10. Laguna MP, de la Rosette JJ (2001) The endoscopic approach to the distal ureter in nephroureterectomy for upper urinary tract tumor. J Urol 166:2017–22
11. Gonzalez CM, Batler RA, Schoor RA, Hairston JC, Nadler RB (2001) A novel endoscopic approach towards resection of the distal ureter with surrounding bladder cuff during hand assisted laparoscopic nephroureterectomy. J Urol 165:483–485
12. Dell'Adami G, Breda G (1976) Transurethral or endoscopic ureterectomy. Eur Urol 2:156–157
13. Shalhav AL, Dunn MD, Portis AJ, Elbahnasy AM, McDougall EM, Clayman RV (2000) Laparoscopic nephroureterectomy for upper tract transitional cell cancer: the Washington University experience. J Urol 163:1100–1104
14. McNeill SA, Chrisofos M, Tolley DA (2000) The long-term outcome after laparoscopic nephroureterectomy: a comparison with open nephroureterectomy. Br J Urol Int 86:619–623
15. Gill IS, Sung GT, Hobart MG, Savage SJ, Meraney AM, Schweizer DK, Klein EA, Novick AC (2000) Laparoscopic radical nephroureterectomy for upper tract transitional cell carcinoma: the Cleveland Clinic experience. J Urol 164:1513–1522

16. Siefman BD, Montie JE, Wolff JS (2000) Prospective comparison between hand-assisted laparoscopic and open surgical nephro-ureterectomy for urothelial cell carcinoma. Urology 57:133–137

17. Ahmed I, Shaikh NA, Kapaidia CR (1998) Track recurrence of renal pelvic transitional cell carcinoma after laparoscopic nephrectomy. Br J Urol 81:319

18. Otani M, Irie S, Tsuji S (1999) Port site metastasis after laparoscopic nephrectomy. Unsuspected transitional cell carcinoma within a tuberculous atrophic kidney. J Urol 162:486–487

19. Jayson M, Sanders H (1998) Increased incidence of serendipitously discovered renal cell carcinoma. Urology 51:203–205

20. Dechet CB, Sebo T, Farrow G, Blute ML, Engen DE, Zincke H (1999) Prospective analysis of intraoperative frozen needle biopsy of solid renal masses in adults. J Urol 162:1282–1285

21. Hafez KS, Fergany AF, Novick AC (1999) Nephron-sparing surgery for localized renal cell carcinoma: impact of tumor size on patient survival, tumor recurrence and TNM staging. J Urol 162:1930–1933

22. Uzzo RG, Novick AC (2001) Nephron sparing surgery for renal tumors: indications, techniques, and outcomes. J Urol 166:6–18

23. Winfield HN, Donovan JF, Godet AS, Clayman RV (1993) Laparoscopic partial nephrectomy: initial case report for benign disease. J Endourol 7:521–526

24. Gill IS, Delworth MG, Munch LC (1994) Laparoscopic retroperitoneal partial nephrectomy. J Urol 152:1539–1542

25. McDougall EM, Elbahnasy AM, Clayman RV (1998) Laparoscopic wedge resection and partial nephrectomy: the Washington University experience and review of literature. J Soc Laparoendosc Surg 2:15–23

26. Janetschek G, Jeschke K, Peschel R, Strohmeyer D, Henning K, Bartsch G (2000) Laparoscopic surgery for stage 1 renal cell carcinoma: radical nephrectomy and wedge resection. Eur Urol 38:131–138

27. Yoshimura K, Okubo K, Ichioka K, Terada N, Matsuta Y, Arai Y (2001) Laparoscopic partial nephrectomy with a microwave tissue coagulator for small renal tumor. J Urol 166:1893–1896

28. Gettman MT, Bishoff JT, Su LM, Chan D, Kavoussi LR, Jarrett TW, Cadeddu JA (2001) Hemostatic laparoscopic partial nephrectomy: initial experience with the radiofrequency coagulation-assisted technique. Urology 58:8–11

29. Gill IS, Desai MM, Kaouk JH, Meraney AM, Murphy DP, Sung GT, Novick AC (2002) Laparoscopic partial nephrectomy for renal tumor: duplicating open surgical techniques. J Urol 167:469–476

30. Janetschek G, Abdelmaksoud A, Bagheri F, Al-Zahrani H, Leeb K, Gschwendtner M (2004) Laparoscopic partial nephrectomy in cold ischemia: renal artery perfusion. J Urol 171:68–71

31. Stephenson RA, King DK, Rohr LR (1996) Renal cryoablation in a canine model. Urology 47:772–776

32. Cozzi PJ, Lynch WJ, Collins S, Vonthethoff L, Morris DL (1997) Renal cryotherapy in a sheep model: a feasibility study. J Urol 157:710–712

33. Gage AA, Baust J (1998) Mechanisms of tissue injury in cryosurgery. Cryobiology 37:171–186

34. Rukstalis DB, Khorsandi M, Garcia FU, Hoenig DM, Cohen JK (2001) Clinical experience with open renal cryoablation. Urology 57:34–39

35. Gill IS, Novick AC, Meraney AM, Chen RN, Hobart MG, Sung GT, Hale J, Schweizer DK, Remer EM (2000) Laparoscopic renal cryoablation in 32 patients. Urology 56:748–53

36. Shingleton WB, Sewell PE (2002) Percutaneous renal cryoablation: 24 and 36-month follow-up [abstract]. J Endourol 16A:133

37. Gervais DA, McGovern FJ, Wood BJ, Goldberg SN, McDougal WS, Mueller PR (2000) Radiofrequency ablation of renal cell carcinoma: early clinical experience. Radiology 217:665–672

38. de Baere T, Kuoch V, Smayra T, Dromain C, Cabrera T, Court B, Roche A (2002) Radio frequency ablation of renal cell carcinoma: preliminary clinical experience. J Urol 167:1961–1964

39. Pavlovich CP, Walther MM, Choyke PL, Pautler SE, Chang R, Linehan WM, Wood BJ (2002) Percutaneous radiofrequency ablation of small renal tumors: initial results. J Urol 167:10–15

40. Lewin JS, Nour SG, Connell CF, Sulman A, Duerk JL, Resnick MI (2002) Follow up findings of a phase II trial of interactive MR-guided radiofrequency thermal ablation of primary kidney tumors [abstract]. Proceedings of 10th Scientific Meeting of the International Society for Magnetic Resonance in Medicine; Honolulu, Hawaii, May 18–24

41. Rendon RA, Kachura JR, Sweet JM, Gertner MR, Sherar MD, Robinette M, Tsihlias J, Trachtenberg J, Sampson H, Jewett MA (2002) The uncertainty of radiofrequency treatment of renal cell carcinoma: findings at immediate and delayed nephrectomy. J Urol 167:1587–1592

42. Matlaga BR, Zagoria RJ, Woodruff RD, Torti FM, Hall MC (2002) Phase II trial of radio frequency ablation of renal cancer: evaluation of the kill zone. J Urol 168:2401–2405

43. Michaels MJ, Rhee HK, Mourtzinos AP, Summerhayes IC, Silverman ML, Libertino JA (2002) Incomplete renal tumor destruction using radio frequency interstitial ablation. J Urol 168:2406–2410

44. Marcovich R, Aldana JP, Morgenstern N, Jacobson AI, Smith AD, Lee BR (2003) Optimal lesion assessment following acute radio frequency ablation of porcine kidney: cellular viability or histopathology? J Urol 170:1370–1374

45. Guillonneau B, Cathelineau X, Barret E, Rozet F, Vallancien G (1999) Laparoscopic radical prostatectomy: technical and early oncological assessment of 40 operations. Eur Urol 36:14–20

46. Guillonneau B, el-Fettouh H, Baumert H, Cathelineau X, Doublet JD, Fromont G, Vallancien G (2003) Laparoscopic radical prostatectomy: oncological evaluation after 1,000 cases at Montsouris Institute. J Urol 169:1261–1266

47. Rassweiler J, Sentker L, Seemann O, Hatzinger M, Rumpelt HJ (2001) Laparoscopic radical prostatectomy with the Heilbronn technique: an analysis of the first 180 cases. J Urol 166:2101–2108

48. Stolzenburg JU, Do M, Rabenalt R, Pfeiffer H, Horn L, Truss MC, Jonas U, Dorschner W (2003) Endoscopic extraperitoneal radical prostatectomy: initial experience after 70 procedures. J Urol 169:2066–2071

49. Long JP, Bahn D, Lee F, Shinohara K, Chinn DO, Macaluso JN Jr (2001) Five-year retrospective multi-institutional pooled analysis of cancer-related outcomes after cryosurgical ablation of the prostate. Urology 57:518–523

50. Thuroff S, Chaussy C, Vallancien G, Wieland W, Kiel HJ, Le Duc A, Desgrandchamps F, De La Rosette JJ, Gelet A (2003) High-intensity focused ultrasound and localized

prostate cancer: efficacy results from the European multicentric study. J Endourol 17:673–677

51. El-Hakim A, Lee BR (2003) Laparoscopic adrenalectomy: when and how. Contemp Urol 15:56–66

52. Luton JP, Cerdas S, Billaud L, Thomas G, Guilhaume B, Bertagna X, Laudat MH, Louvel A, Chapuis Y, Blondeau P, et al (1990) Clinical features of adrenocortical carcinoma, prognostic factors, and the effect of mitotane therapy. N Engl J Med 322:1195–1201

53. Lam K, Lo C (2002) Metastatic tumours of the adrenal glands: a 30-year experience in a teaching hospital. Clin Endocrinol (Oxf) 56:95–101

54. Heniford B, Arca M, Walsh R, Gill I (1999) Laparoscopic adrenalectomy for cancer. Semin Surg Oncol 16:293–306

55. Belldegrun A, Hussain S, Seltzer S, Loughlin K, Gittes R, Richie J (1986) Incidentally discovered mass of the adrenal gland. Surg Gynecol Obstet 163:203–208

56. Janetschek G, Hobisch A, Peschel R, Hittmair A, Bartsch G (2000) Laparoscopic retroperitoneal lymph node dissection for clinical stage I nonseminomatous testicular carcinoma: long-term outcome J Urol 163:1793–1796

57. Bhayani SB, Ong A, Oh WK, Kantoff PW, Kavoussi LR (2003) Laparoscopic retroperitoneal lymph node dissection for clinical stage I nonseminomatous germ cell testicular cancer: a long-term update. Urology 62:324–327

58. Palese MA, Su LM, Kavoussi LR (2002) Laparoscopic retroperitoneal lymph node dissection after chemotherapy. Urology 60:130–134

59. Janetschek G, Hobisch A, Hittmair A, Holtl L, Peschel R, Bartsch G (1999) Laparoscopic retroperitoneal lymphadenectomy after chemotherapy for stage IIB nonseminomatous testicular carcinoma. J Urol 161:477–481

60. United States Renal Data System. *USRDS 2003 Annual Data Reprot*. Bethesda, MD: National Institute of Diabetes and Digestive and Kidney Diseases, National Institutes of Health (NIH), DHHS; 2003. Available at www.usrds.org.

61. El-Hakim A, Chertin B, Marcovich R, Lee BR, Weiss GH, Smith AD (2004) Adjuvant bacillus Calmette-Guérin therapy after endoscopic treatment of upper tract transitional cell carcinoma: first proof of efficacy. J Urol 171 (Supp): Absract 1760, 465

Surgical Robots and Three-Dimensional Displays for Computer-Aided Surgery

TAKEYOSHI DOHI

Summary. Surgery in the 21st century will use advanced technologies such as surgical robots, three-dimensional medical imaging, computer graphics, computer simulation technology, and others. Three-dimensional medical imaging for surgical operations provides surgeons with advanced vision. A surgical robot provides surgeons with an advanced hand, but it is not a machine to perform the same action of a surgeon using scissors or scalpels. Recently, two new systems were developed in Japan: an advanced vision system called integral videography (IV), which can project a full-color three-dimensional video image in real three-dimensional space, and a novel robotic endoscopic system using two wedge prisms at the tip, which can observe a wide area without moving or bending the endoscope. As an advanced hand, a high-safety navigation robot of the laparoscope and a forceps manipulator with a bending mechanism have also been developed in Japan. The advanced vision and hands available to surgeons are creating new surgical fields in the 21st century: minimally invasive surgery, noninvasive surgery, virtual reality microsurgery, telesurgery, fetal surgery, neuroinformatics surgery, and others.

Keywords. Computer-aided surgery, Advanced vision, Advanced hand, Surgical robot, Integral videography

Introduction

Surgical operations have developed with the skillful use of the surgeon's hands and eyes. Therefore, it is very difficult to apply advanced technologies to surgical operations. To develop the new surgical fields of minimally invasive surgery, noninvasive surgery, virtual reality microsurgery, telesurgery, fetal surgery, neuroinformatics surgery, and others in the 21st century, it is necessary to use various

Graduate School of Information Science and Technology, Department of Mechano-Informatics, The University of Tokyo, 7-3-1 Hongo, Bunkyo-ku, Tokyo 113-8656, Japan

15

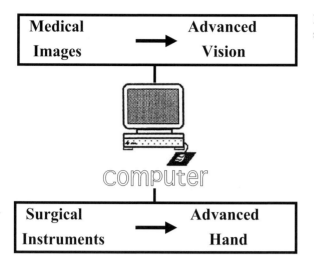

Fɪɢ. 1. Computer-aided surgery

advanced technologies with surgical robots, three-dimensional medical images, etc., based on computer technology. This new surgical field is called computer-aided surgery (CAS) [1]. The reconstructed three-dimensional medical images provide the most recognizable information for medical doctors and advanced visualization for surgeons. Surgical robots function as advanced hands for surgeons. The advanced vision and hands available to surgeons are creating a new surgical environment (Fig. 1).

Advanced Vision

Usually, medical images in a surgical field are used mainly for diagnosis before and after the operation. Computer graphics technology visualizes the three-dimensional structure of organs, vessels, and tumors using information from X-ray computed tomography (CT), magnetic resonance imaging (MRI), echography, and so on. The main fields of research on three-dimensional medical images in CAS are the acquisition system, the reconstruction method, multi-modality matching, and three-dimensional display.

Three-Dimensional Display

There are three kinds of display methods for three-dimensional image:
Pseudo-three-dimensional display. Basically, this display is a two-dimensional display. A stereoscopic feeling is obtained by rotating a three-dimensional model on a two-dimensional display. As three-dimensional models, there are the voxel model and the surface model.

Binocular stereoscopic display. This method uses two two-dimensional images for binocular vision. The feeling of depth is provided mainly by binocular parallax and convergence. However, the absolute three-dimensional position cannot be given. Since observation by this method is not physiological, observation for a long time causes visual fatigue. As displays of this method, there are a stereoscope, a parallax stereogram, and a three-dimensional lenticular sheet.

True three-dimensional display. The true three-dimensional display produces a three-dimensional image in real three-dimensional space. As displays of this method, there are holography, integral photography (IP), and volume graph based on the principle of IP. Since observation by this method is physiological, this observation does not cause visual fatigue. Absolute three-dimensional positions and motion parallax are given. IP projects three-dimensional models using a two-dimensional lens array called a "fly's eye lens (FEL)" and a photographic film. Recently, a computer-generated IP called integral videography (IV) has been developed by FEL and color liquid crystal display (Figs. 2 and 3) [2]. IV can display full-color video. The volume graph and IV give absolute three-dimensional positions and they are much simpler than holography, which uses interference of laser light. They can project the reconstructed 3D model at geometrically exact position in internal cavity with relatively minimal computation and engineering effort. Therefore they are very suitable for three-dimensional display for surgical navigation.

Table 1 compares the binocular stereoscopic image and the true three-dimensional image for surgery.

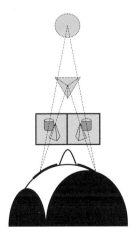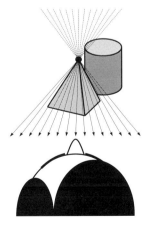

FIG. 2. Binocular stereoscopic display (*left*) and true three-dimensional display (*right*)

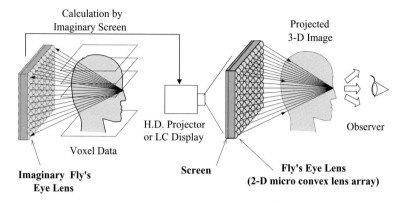

FIG. 3. Integral videography. *HD*, high definition; *LC*, liquid cristal

TABLE 1. Comparison between binocular stereoscopic image and true three-dimensional (3-D) image for surgery

		Binocular	True 3-D
Image	Fineness	Excellent	Good
	Processing	Simple	Complicated
	Special glasses	Necessary	Unnecessary
3-D Rec.	Parallax	Fixed	Physiological
	Convergence	Fixed	Physiological
	Accommodation	Fixed	Physiological
	3-D position	Only feeling	Absolute position
	Visual fatigue	Inevitable	Free
	Number of observes	Limited	Not so limited
Suitable application		Intraoperative	Percutaneous navigator

Advanced Hand [3]

The typical advanced hand for surgeons is a surgical robot. The surgical robot is one of the medical robots and has the problems common to medical robots. Medical robots are quite different from industrial robots in the following four aspects:

These robots contact the human body directly.

The combination of surgical maneuvering differs by cases; modifying the combination to adopt to patients' condition is necessary.

When these robots are used in practice, trial movement or redoing is not allowed.

These robots can be operated easily even if the operator is not a specialist.

Safety of Medical Robot

Safety of industrial robot is guaranteed by maintaining the gap between the robot and the human. This approach is not applicable to medical robot where robots contact the patient (human.) Therefore, the safety measure should be taken from both software and hardware aspects in medical robotics, where the measure is taken mostly hardware configuration in industrial robotics.

Medical robots must be designed so that a user can cope easily when the robot causes trouble. There are four kinds of emergency actions, and which action to adopt differs according to the kind of surgical robot:

Stop in the position where an emergency happened (= Freeze).
Move to the original or specified position automatically.
Escape to the safe position automatically in case of emergency, then to arbitrary position after emergency.
Move to the arbitrary position manually.

Classification of Surgical Robots

An advanced hand for a surgeon is one of the medical instruments, and it is called a surgical robot or therapeutic robot. There are two kinds of surgical robots for CAS, the navigation robot and the treatment robot. Three-dimensional medical images during an operation by surgical robots are very important.

Navigation robot. Navigation robots are percutaneous needle punctures, cannulations, and others. Safety and minimally invasive navigation to a diseased part are very important to achieve a good result from a surgical operation. It is especially important for this robot to access the complicated parts that cannot be accessed directly by the surgeon.

Treatment robot. These robots are required to have functions of cutting, resection, exfoliation, suture, ligation, and others. However, these functions should be designed in the mechanism, which is suitable for mechanical operation. The robot should be designed specifically to achieve these surgical maneuvering instead of re-using general purpose robot.

Principles of Design of Medical Robots

Surgical operations have developed with the skillful use of the surgeon's hands and eyes. Many surgical operations are not suitable for performance by a machine. Moreover, a machine that performs the same action as a surgeon cannot perform treatment better than a surgeon. Therefore, a surgical robot does not just imitate the surgeon's action, but it must be designed in consideration of the following points:

It should be designed corresponding to the purpose of treatment.
Robot should be designed to best achieve the targeted surgical maneuvering which otherwise is less effective by manual maneuvering.

It should provide better treatment than the current treatment provided by the surgeon's eyes and hands.

It should make the most of the current knowledge and experience of the surgeon.

Development Situation in Japan

Navigator of a Laparoscope

As an application of robotics to laparoscopic surgery, a navigation robot system for laparoscopy with a CCD camera has been developed. It is required that this kind of navigation robot should be safe at all times. It is especially important that neither the abdominal wall nor the internal organs of the patient be damaged. This problem is solved by combining a planar five-bar linkage mechanism and a fixed ball joint placed on the abdominal wall (Fig. 4) [4]. In Japan, it has been developed and marketed under the brand name Naviot. This navigator fulfills the important conditions of the surgical robot. It has the following features as compared with other navigators:

There is no danger of damaging the abdominal wall and internal organs.
The operation area on the abdomen is very wide.
The drive section and the five-bar linkage mechanism section can separate easily.
Washing and sterilization of the five-bar linkage section are very easy.
Operation by the surgeon himself or herself is very easy.

A novel robotic endoscope system has also been developed. It can be used to observe a wide area without moving or bending the endoscope. The system con-

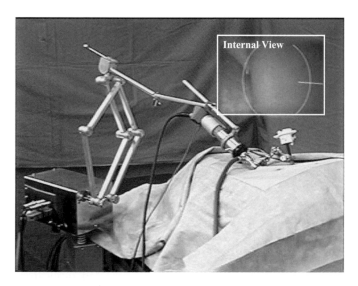

Fig. 4. Naviot navigator of laparascope

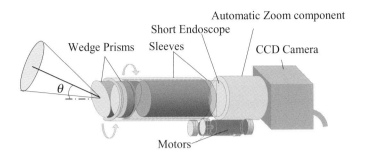

simple and small mechanism

Fig. 5. Construction of the wide-range endoscope system using wedge prisms. *CCD*, charge-coupled device

sists of a laparoscope with zoom facility and two wedge prisms at the tip (Fig. 5) [5]. This new concept produces the following excellent characteristics. First, it can change the field of view even in a small space. Second, it is safe because it avoids the possibility of hitting the internal organs. Finally, because it does not require a large mechanism for manipulation of the endoscope, it does not obstruct the surgeon's operation. During evaluation, it was confirmed that the range of view and levels of image deformation were acceptable for clinical use.

In order to keep a treatment space in the abdomen, a gasless method for lifting the abdominal wall by subcutaneous wiring has been developed in Japan [6]. This method has several merits compared with the pneumoperitoneum method. When robot technology is applied for laparoscopic surgery, the abdominal wall-lifting method is far better than the pneumoperitoneum method.

Stereotaxic Surgery

Stereotaxic surgery is a kind of neurosurgery that requires precise positioning of the surgical apparatus, using predetermined location information. According to information on the position of the tumor (or any target) in the brain obtained by X-ray CT (or MRI) sliced images, the coordinates of the instruments are set manually, and a cannulation needle is inserted into the tumor. We have developed a cannulation manipulator to cooperate with the CAS system. This manipulator has 6 degrees of freedom. The needle is inserted to the target position according to the precalculated direction by specifying the parameters of the freedoms. All components of the manipulator are designed to fit the size of the opening of the CT scanner. The manipulator has a safety-oriented design and compactness. When the CAS system is used for cannulation of the needle to the brain tumor, the optimal path of the needle toward the tumor is calculated so as not to damage the functional area of the brain and the major brain vessels. The manipulator inserts the needle to the tumor through the planned path. This manipulator can also be used for X-ray CT-guided stereotaxic surgery.

Ultrasound computed tomography (USCT) for neurosurgery was also developed in 1995 [7]. USCT reconstructs arbitrary planes from multiple scans taken during rotation of the probe.

A three-dimensional overlay system for neurosurgery called the volumegraph has been developed (Fig. 6). The volumegraph is a sheet that has recorded a three-dimensional image before the operation, and this image is observed without special glasses. In September 1996, the first operation using this system was successfully performed at Tokyo Women's Medical College. With this system, the medical doctors can confirm the target position before opening the head, and it is easy to decide the access point and the opening area of the head [8]. The integral videography system is now used for neurosurgery [9].

Stem-Cell Harvesting Manipulator [10]

A stem-cell harvesting manipulator system has been developed in my laboratory. This device efficiently harvests bone marrow for transplantation with the use of a newly developed passive flexible drilling unit and suction mechanism. The device reduces the invasiveness of bone marrow harvesting by collecting stem cells from the iliac bone with minimal punctures and by reducing opera-

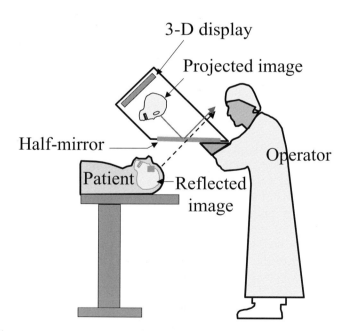

FIG. 6. Navigation system by superimposition

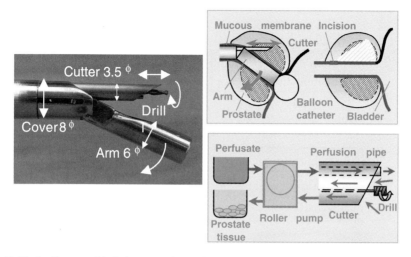

FIG. 7. End-effector with 3 degrees of freedom: arm, cutter, and drill

tion time and contamination by T-cells. The device is inserted into the medullary space from the iliac crest and aspirates the bone marrow while an end mill on the tip of the drilling unit drills through the cancellous bone to create a curved path (Fig. 7). In vitro and in vivo pig studies showed that the device can be inserted into the medullary space of the pig iliac bone and used to harvest about six times as much bone marrow per puncture as the conventional aspiration method. The studies also showed that the device can generate higher and longer negative pressure than the aspiration method. The device, when applied in clinical study, will reduce invasiveness by harvesting a denser graft from a wider area of the iliac bone compared with the conventional aspiration method, although minimal puncturing is required.

Transurethral Resection of the Prostate (TURP) [11]

Currently, transurethral resection of the prostate (TURP) is the gold-standard treatment and the most common surgical procedure for benign prostatic hyperplasia (BPH). However, damage to the mucous membrane of the urethra and extended surgery lead to complications. In order to resolve these problems, we have proposed a new prostatectomy and developed a TURP manipulator that has a prostate displacement mechanism and a continuous perfusion-resection mechanism (Fig. 8). This manipulator has 3 degrees of freedom: bending an arm, translating a cutter, and rotating a drill at the end effector. The arm enters and bends the prostate; the cutter is then inserted into the enlarged prostate, the drill cuts the enlarged tissue into small pieces, and a pump removes them by suction. The mechanism can resect the prostate quickly without damaging the mucous membrane.

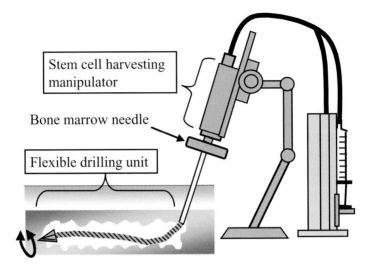

Fɪɢ. 8. Concept of the stem-cell harvesting manipulator

Forceps Manipulator with a Bending Mechanism [12]

A new endoscopic hand-held forceps manipulator for endoscopic surgery using two bending mechanisms by multislider linkage mechanisms to achieve high mechanical performance and applicability has been developed in our laboratory. One bending mechanism is for horizontal plane bending, and the other is for vertical plane bending, enabling 2 degrees of freedom of independent motion between ±90° and +90°. To realize the bending of the top of the forceps, the multislider linkage mechanism is superior to the wire-driven mechanism. The bending mechanism consists of three outer frames, two rotating joints, and two sliding linkages for drive and restraint. Two pin joints can each rotate ±45°, enabling rotation of ±90°. Rotation of the joint is accomplished by pulling or pushing the adjacent element by sliding linkage in order (Fig. 9). An in vivo experiment showed that this manipulator performed endoscopic surgical tasks under the pneumoperitoneum and was confirmed as easy to operate.

Conclusions

Applications of three-dimensional images and robotics in medicine are widespread in clinical use. As a new concept of robot systems in medicine, it is necessary to integrate with three-dimensional imaging technologies. By this integration, surgical treatments so far impossible or difficult will be enabled or facilitated. Medical robots and three-dimensional medical images provide advanced hands and vision for surgeons; in the 21st century, these new devices for surgeons will develop new surgical fields, such as virtual reality microsurgery, telesurgery,

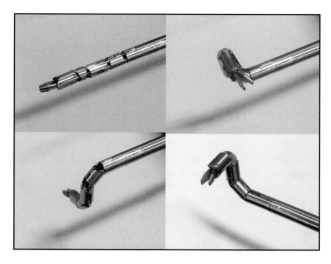

FIG. 9. Multi-degree of freedom (DOF) end-effector with 2-DOF bending mechanism and 1-DOF forceps mechanism

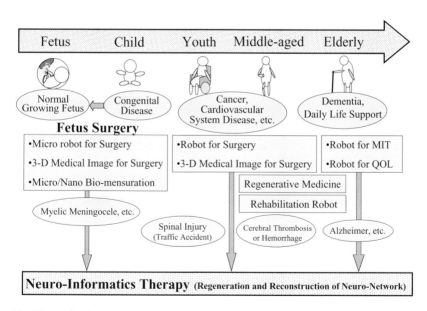

FIG. 10. New robotic surgery fields for disabled persons. *MIT*, Minimally invasive therapy; *QOL*, quality of life

fetal surgery, neuroinformatics surgery, and others (Fig. 10). However, engineers who develop medical instruments should be reminded that the clinical environment is quite different from the industrial one, and should develop clinically oriented devices instead of just applying industrial robots.

References

1. Dohi T, Ohta, Y, Suzuki M, Chinzei K, Horiuchi T, Hashimoto D, Tsuzuki M (1990) Computer aided surgery system (CAS) -development of surgical simulation and planning system with three dimensional graphic reconstruction. 1st Conference on Visualization in Biomedical Computing, IEEE, 458
2. Nakajima S, Kobayashi E, Orita S, Masamune K, Sakuma I, Dohi T (1999) Development of a 3-D display system to project 3-D image in a real 3-D space. Proceedings of 3D Image Conference '99, 49–54, Tokyo, Japan
3. Dohi T, Hata N, Miyata K, Hashimoto D, Takakura K, Chinzei K, Yamauchi Y (1995) Robotics in computer aided surgery system. J Computer Aided Surg 1(1):4–10
4. Kobayashi E, Masamune K, Suzuki M, Dohi T, Hashimoto D (1996) Development on a laparoscope navigator using a planar five-bar linkage. Proceedings of 5th Conference of Japan Society of Computer Aided Surgery, 77–78
5. Kobayashi E, Masamune K, Sakuma I, Dohi T (2000) A wide-angle view endoscope system using wedge prisms. Medical Image Computing and Computer-Assisted Intervention-MICCAI 2000, 661–668
6. Hashimoto D, Nayeem SA, Hoshino T (1995) Advanced techniques in gasless laparoscopic surgery. World Scientific Publishing, Singapore
7. Hata N, Suzuki M, Dohi T, Takakura K, Iseki H, Kawabatake H, Yamauchi Y, Umaki K (1994) Ultrasound CT, Image technology & information display, 94-OCT, 1194–1198
8. Yamane F, Iseki H, Masutani Y, Iwahara M, Nishi Y, Kawamura H, Tanikawa T, Kawabatake H, Taira T, Suzuki M, Dohi T, Takakura K (1995) Three-dimensional image guided navigation with function of augmented reality. Proceedings of 4th Conference of Japan Society of Computer Aided Surgery, 99–100, Tokyo, Japan.
9. Liao H, Nakajima S, Iwahara M, Hata N, Sakuma I, Dohi T (2002) Real-time 3D image-guided navigation system based on integral videography. Proceedings of SPIE Vol 4615, pp 36–44, San Jose, California
10. Ohashi K, Hata N, Matsumura T, Ogata T, Yahagi N, Sakuma I, Dohi T (2003) Stem cell harvesting device with passive flexible drilling unit for bone marrow transplantation. IEEE Trans Rob Autom 19:810–817
11. Hashimoto R, Kim D, Hata N, Dohi T (2003) A transurethral prostate resection manipulator for minimal damage to mucous membrane. Proceedings of the 6th Annual International Conference on Medical Image Computing and Computer Assisted Intervention, MICCAI 2003, LNCS 2878. Springer, pp 149–157, Montreal, Canada
12. Yamashita H, Kim D, Hata N, Dohi T (2003) Multi-slider linkage mechanism for endoscopic forceps manipulator. Proceedings of the 2003 IEEE/RSJ International Conference on Intelligent Robots and Systems (IROS 2003), Vol 3, pp 2577–2582, Las Vegas, Nevada, U.S.A.

Robot-Assisted (Da Vinci) Urologic Surgery: An Emerging Frontier

ASHOK K. HEMAL and MANI MENON

Summary. Robotic urologic surgery is an interesting and new development in the field of urology that has tremendous possibilities for progress in the future. Reports from various centers worldwide of complex urologic procedures in humans performed with robotic assistance have documented their safety, efficacy, efficiency, and feasibility. This review attempts to define the incorporation of robotics into laparoscopic urologic surgery and also reflects on our experience with over 900 cases of robotic surgery. Most of the recent reports pertaining to robotic surgery have been in the domain of localized cancer of the prostate (radical prostatectomy), bladder cancer (radical cystectomy and urinary diversion for muscle-invasive bladder cancer), kidney surgery (nephrectomy, donor nephrectomy, and pyeloplasty), and adrenal surgery. There are also reports in other areas of urology such as male infertility.

Keywords. Robotics, Urology, Prostate, Bladder, Kidney, Adrenal

Introduction

Laparoscopic urologic surgery (LUS) has been on the horizon for over a decade and has benefited patients in terms of lower morbidity, less pain, shorter hospital stay, less discomfort, and excellent cosmesis with minimal invasion [1]. LUS obviates the morbidity in terms of pain, discomfort, and disability that is often associated with open surgery due to the process of gaining access to the specific organ or region of interest, as opposed to the actual procedure itself. However, in laparoscopic surgery coordinated tactile feedback is significantly lost, and the surgeon's actions are further compromised by limitations in the movement of the instruments and loss of depth perception due to two-dimensional vision. Further, a human assistant is needed to control the camera. Thus, the impedi-

Vattikuti Urology Institute, Henry Ford Hospital, 2799 West Grand Boulevard, Detroit, MI 48202, USA

ment to widespread use of laparoscopy in urology has been twofold: the technical demands of laparoscopy coupled with the complexity of urologic procedures. Consequently, advanced LUS is limited to relatively few experts and centers worldwide [2, 3]. The addition of robotic assistance may help to overcome some of the challenges posed by the limitations of laparoscopy. Robotic assistance appears as a natural expansion of traditional laparoscopy, offering the inherent advantages of minimally invasive surgery while additionally improving the surgeon's ability to perform technically challenging operations [3, 4]. At the time of writing, we have performed over 900 robotic urologic procedures at our center, including commonly performed robotic radical prostatectomy.

Development of Robotic and Robot-Assisted Laparoscopic Urologic Surgery

Robots were first used in humans to perform transurethral resection for the treatment of benign hyperplasia of the prostate at Imperial College in London [5]. A second-generation robot was also developed by the same team for resection of the prostate gland and was named "Probot." The detailed history of the development of the robot has been described in the literature [6]. The robotic system aids in dexterity enhancement, precision localization, and manipulation.

Technologically, the robotic system can be categorized into three types:

Autonomous: the preoperative plan controls the manipulator.
Supervisory: the computer accurately guides the surgeon to perform the surgery.
Teleoperated: input devices are under the surgeon's control from a remote control robotic console.

The other way to classify a robot is as active or passive. A passive robot system has been used in the past to hold the camera during laparoscopy; it can also be used for visceral retraction. An active robot performs the task by actually moving the tools. Three such systems are available: AESOP (automated endoscopic system for optimal positioning) (Computer motion, Goleta, CA, USA); FIP endoarm and EndoWrist (Intuitive Surgical Inc., Sunnyvale, CA, USA); and the master-slave manipulator system, in which the operator manipulates a "master" device from a surgical console using a type of joystick whose movements are translated to comparable movements in the "slave" robot performing the task.

da Vinci Robotic Technology

The da Vinci robotic system is a sophisticated master-slave robot that has three multijoint robotic arms. In recent model a fourth arm is available, although its usefulness has not yet been clearly defined. The central arm controls the camera, and the other two arms control the articulated instruments. Currently, two lenses (0 and 30 degrees) are available. The surgeon controls the movement of these arms from a remote station, a foot pedal controls the camera movements, and two finger-controlled handles (masters) located in a mobile console manipulate the robotic arms that carry the articulating robotic instruments. The three-dimensional, 10–15 times magnified vision, the seven degrees of freedom of movement, the scaling of movements, and the articulating robotic endowrist (which allows mimicking of the surgeon's hand movements) permit fine dissection in confined spaces and ease in dealing with vascular structures and organs located near the vital structures.

Ergonomics for Surgeons

In LUS, excessive force and torque on sensitive areas of the surgeon's palm and fingers can lead to unnecessary fatigue, discomfort, and temporary neuropraxia. Robotic assistance is ergonomically excellent for the operating surgeon, as it provides ideal posture and an optimal grip on the manipulating instruments and prevents fatigue by allowing the surgeon to sit in a chair at the console.

Robotics (da Vinci-Assisted) in Urologic Surgery

Table 1 depicts what is on the horizon for robotics in laparoscopic urology at this point in time. For each application, the question is being asked, "How do these new techniques compare with the current standard open techniques"? Most surgical procedures currently being performed can be classified as ablative or reconstructive. Ablative procedures in urology may be either diagnostic (e.g., lymph node dissection) or therapeutic (e.g., nephrectomy, adrenalectomy), whereas reconstructive procedures are ureteropelvic junction repair (pyeloplasty), partial nephrectomy, etc. The other group of procedures utilizes both components (ablative and reconstructive); the most commonly performed operation in this group is robot-assisted radical prostatectomy. The important procedures that are currently being performed are briefly described below.

Robot (da Vinci)-Assisted Radical Prostatectomy for Prostate Cancer

Radical anatomic retropubic prostatectomy is the most commonly performed procedure for surgical treatment of localized carcinoma of the prostate [7]. Laparoscopic radical prostatectomy is a minimally invasive technique for surgical management of adenocarcinoma of the prostate [8]. Despite tremendous efforts to make this procedure easy and reproducible, it is still lengthy and technically challenging. It has the benefit of decreased invasiveness, which translates into less hospital stay, less pain, and earlier resumption of normal activities for the patient [9–13]. The greatest potential advantage of laparoscopic prostatectomy is the excellent magnified view of the operative field. This enables better

TABLE 1. Current status of robotic surgery in urology

Ablative	Reconstructive	Miscellaneous
Kidney	Prostate	Donor nephrectomy
Nephrectomy	Robot-assisted radical	Renal transplantation
Nephroureterectomy	prostatectomy	Urogynecology
Partial nephrectomy	(most common procedure)	Bladder neck
Radical nephrectomy	Sural nerve grafting	suspension for
Radical nephroureterectomy	Retropubic prostatectomy for	stress urinary
Adrenal	benign prostatic hyperplasia	incontinence
Adrenalectomy	Bladder	Male infertility
	Laparoscopic radical	Vasovasostomy
	cystectomy with creation of	Vasoepididymostomy
	orthotopic neobladder or	
	ileal conduit.	
	Diverticulectomy	
	Boari's flap creation and	
	ureteroneocystostomy	
	Pyeloplasty for ureteropelvic-	
	junction obstruction	
	Ureterolysis for	
	retroperitoneal fibrosis	
	Ureteroureterostomy	

dissection with decreased blood loss. However, laparoscopic prostatectomy is still not very popular because of limitations of the laparoscopic procedure, the long, steep learning curve, and the loss of dexterity and maneuverability. For surgeons who do not have advanced laparoscopic skills, the most difficult step in the procedure is suturing in reconstructive urologic surgery such as vesico-urethral suturing in Medical prostatectomy vesicourethral suturing. Many of these disadvantages can be overcome with robotic assistance, which allows the surgeon to dissect, suture, and tie knots in a relaxed manner remote from the patient. Various scientists reported on their initial experience with robotic radical prostatectomy [14–17]. However, it was not until large series emerged from different centers that interest was rekindled worldwide [18–22]. The robot arms respond to movements of the surgeon's hands, allowing them to mimic the steps of open surgery. The largest experience in the world has been obtained at the Vattikuti Urology Institute, Henry Ford Hospital, where over 800 robotic radical prostatectomies have been performed up to this time. In 2003 alone, 344 operations were performed with the Vattikuti Institute Prostatectomy (VIP) technique.

Vattikuti Institute Prostatectomy (VIP) Technique

At our center, laparoscopic radical prostatectomy was initiated in October 2000, and the first robot-assisted radical prostatectomy was performed in November 2000. A variety of modifications were introduced subsequently. The details of the development of this structured program have been published [3]. Our current VIP technique was developed step-by-step over a period of time, based on knowledge of conventional and laparoscopic radical prostatectomy with the technical advantages of robotic assistance. We have previously described the technique [23, 24]. We perform robotic radical prostatectomy using a six-port approach and the Da Vinci Surgical System (Intuitive Surgical, Sunnyvale, CA, USA).

The salient steps of the technique are the following:

Step I. Entering the space of Retzius. Pneumoperitoneum is created by the standard technique, and ports are placed in the fashion described by us in previous publications. The bladder is taken down from the anterior abdominal wall by making parallel incisions lateral to the medial umbilical ligaments on both sides and subsequently joining these horizontally in the midline. Care is taken not to get into the bladder. Usually this part of the dissection is easy, as it involves dividing loose areolar, fatty tissue and mainly less vascular structures. Once the retropubic space is entered, the dissection needs to be very careful and gentle, since teasing off fatty tissues may lead to unwarranted oozing. The superficial dorsal veins are fulgurated, and fat is cleared from the anterior surface of the prostate so that the shiny endopelvic fascia can be seen laterally.

Step II. Incision of the endopelvic fascia. The endopelvic fascia is entered at the point where it reflects over the pelvic side wall, and the levator ani muscle is gently teased away to expose the lateral surface of the prostate. The incision is then extended in an anteromedial direction towards the apex of the prostate to expose the dorsal vein, urethra, and striated urethral sphincter. Most of the dissection is done bluntly near the apex of the prostate to expose the urethra, which is freed at the apex of the prostate from underlying neurovascular bundle bilaterally.

Step III. Control of dorsal vein complex. The dorsal vein complex and striated sphincter are very closely associated, and meticulous control of bleeding helps in the precise division of the urethra and sphincter, which in turn helps in anastomosis and consequently in an early return of continence. Even a minor bleed may jeopardize the surgeon's vision, especially in robot-assisted radical prostatectomy. A 0-vicryl stitch on a CT-1 needle is used to ligate the deep dorsal vein. The needle is passed underneath the dorsal vein from one side to the other, grasped from the contralateral side, and then passed above the dorsal vein complex and underneath the puboprostatic ligaments; thus, ligaments are not included in the suture, which permits a tight knot. We also employ a traction suture through the anterior commissure of the prostate, and the ends of this stitch are cut somewhat long. This suture helps the assistant to retract the prostate during the dissection and division of the bladder neck.

Step IV. Division of the bladder neck. The bladder neck is identified with the help of the shiny, smooth pad of fat that lies at the prostatovesical junction. Care is taken while dividing the bladder neck to maintain a clear detrusor margin, which helps during the urethrovesical anastomosis. Reconstruction of the bladder neck prior to anastomosis is rarely required, except in the instance of a large bladder neck opening due to a large median lobe or a large prostate. If necessary, after completion of the urethrovesical anastomosis, the remaining open bladder neck is reconstructed with interrupted sutures of 3-0 vicryl to approximate its full-thickness muscularis and mucosa.

Step V. Nerve-sparing. Standard nerve preservation is not very difficult in robotic radical prostatectomy. However, when we wish to preserve the nerves in the lateral pelvic fascia, which we call the "veil of Aphrodite" (this veil contains the accessory nerves on the lateral prostatic surface), the prostatic fascia is incised on the anterolateral surface of the prostate, close to the previously placed traction suture, anterior and parallel to the neurovascular bundles. The lateral pelvic fascia is methodically separated from the prostatic surface using a combination of blunt and sharp dissection with the articulated, round-tip scissors. At the end of the dissection, the preserved lateral pelvic fascia is seen like a veil of tissue that extends from the prostatovesical to the prostatourethral junction, the "veil of Aphrodite."

Step VI. Division of the urethra. Next, using the EndoWrist round-tip scissors, the dorsal vein complex is divided down to the urethra. An attempt is made to get a good urethral stump, although not at the cost of increasing the rate of positive apical margins.

Step VII. Vesicourethral anastomosis. The vesicourethral anastomosis is performed with a 0-degree laparoscope. For this part of the surgery, to begin with, we have an EndoWrist Long-Tip Forceps in the left hand and an EndoWrist Large Needle Driver in the right hand. The long-tip forceps helps in holding the bladder neck in an atraumatic fashion and also in cinching down the bladder after a couple of sutures. The vesicourethal anastomosis is performed mucosa-to-mucosa in a choreographed sequence as described by van Velthoven et al. and by us earlier [25, 26]. It is begun hemicircumferentially towards the left side, using the needle of the dyed end, by passing the needle outside in at the 4- or 5-o'clock position on the bladder neck and inside out on the urethra. After two or three throws on the urethra and three or four throws on the bladder to create an adequate posterior base, the bladder is cinched down against the knot of the sutures lying on the posterior surface of the bladder. At this point, the long-tip forceps is replaced with an EndoWrist large Needle Driver. The anastomosis is continued in a clockwise fashion up to the 9 o'clock position on the bladder. The suture is then turned into the bladder in such a way that it runs inside out on the bladder and outside in on the urethra to continue further up to the 11 or 12 o'clock position. Then the suture (dyed) is pulled cranially towards the left lateral side of the pelvis and maintained under traction by an assistant. Subsequently, the anastomosis is started on the right side of the urethra with the undyed end, passing it outside in on the urethra and then inside out on the bladder, from the point where the anastomosis was started and continuing in an anticlockwise fashion up to the point where the other suture is met. The needle of the dyed end is cut off, and the free dyed end and the undyed ends are tied together with multiple knots. The urethral catheter is used as a guide in showing the urethral mucosa during the anastomosis, and it is advanced into the bladder before tying the knot. The patency of the urethrovesical anastomosis is tested with instillation of 150 to 200 ml of water, and then the balloon of the Foley's catheter is inflated. A drain is used only in cases where the anastomosis is not watertight.

Outcome Analysis

It is very important to define the primary outcome and the relative merits of VIP with open and laparoscopic prostatectomy. To address some of these issues, a comparison was conducted of 200 cases of VIP with 100 cases of gold-standard retropubic radical prostatectomy in terms of oncological completeness and preservation of erectile function. Undoubtedly, VIP had the clear edge in terms of less blood loss, less postoperative pain, excellent anatomical anastomosis leading to early achievement of continence, visually superb preservation of neurovascular bundle, shorter hospital stay, and cosmesis [27].

In another report on the outcome of 500 cases of robotic radical prostatectomy, it was observed that the incorporation of robotics resulted in better surgical outcomes in comparison with standard and laparoscopic radical prosta-tectomy [28]. There are no differences between the procedures in oncological completeness, margin positivity rate, and surgical outcome, in terms of providing excellent anastomosis and preservation of the neurovascular bundle with superb cosmesis. The preservation of neurovascular bundles and perfect anastomosis translates into achievement of early continence and return of erectile function in our experience. Currently, 96% of our patients achieve continence at 3 months.

Comments

Robotic assistance allowed us to perform excellent anatomical dissection due to excellent visualization, precision, accuracy, and dexterity of the robot by scaling and filtering of hand movements. However, it does require the skill, experience, and wisdom of the surgeon in using the robot flawlessly for the execution of complex surgical maneuvers, particularly during division of the bladder neck, dissection of the vas deferens-seminal vesicle complex, dissection of the preserva-tion of neurovascular bundles, division of the urethra, and vesico-urethral anastomosis, which are often considered difficult steps.

Bladder Cancer: Robot-Assisted Radical Cystectomy and Urinary Diversion

Radical cystectomy is the accepted gold standard for the treatment of muscle-invasive bladder cancer [29]. With the advent of laparoscopy in urology, differ-ent procedures have been described with clear benefits, and the feasibility of laparoscopic radical cystectomy has also been described in various reports

[30–32]. Nevertheless, the inherent limitations of laparoscopic technique result in longer operative time, blood loss, and complications, and the creation of urinary diversion is an extremely difficult step. The potential advantages of robotics assistance can be utilized in this type of urooncologic procedure. After gaining experience in robotic radical prostatectomy, we performed robot-assisted radical cystoprostatectomy (RRCP) in men with bladder cancer, and both standard and uterus-preserving techniques in women with bladder cancer [33]. Usually, RRCP and urinary diversion were carried out using a three-step approach described by us [34], which essentially consists of a complete pelvic lymphadenectomy and cystoprostatectomy utilizing a posterior technique and removal of the specimen through small midline incision, exteriorization of the bowel through this incision and creation of a neobladder extracorporeally, and finally repositioning of the neobladder in the pelvis with closure of the incision to complete the urethroneovesical anastomosis with robotic assistance after reinstallation. In women, pelvic lymphadenectomy, cystectomy, urethrectomy, hysterectomy, salpingo-oophorectomy, and excision of the rim of the vagina are performed if there is suspicion of involvement of the cervix or uterus or extensive disease; otherwise, the operation is performed to preserve the urethra, uterus, ovaries, and vagina. Robotic assistance allowed precise and rapid removal of the bladder with minimal blood loss. Creation of the orthotopic neobladder through the incision utilized to deliver the cystectomy specimen reduces the operative time and cost. Only two case series and one case report of robotic radical cystectomy using the da Vinci system have been published in the English literature [35].

Kidney and Adrenal

First, the feasibility of robot-assisted nephrectomy and adrenalectomy was reported in the pig [36]. Subsequently, the use of robotics has been demonstrated in nephrectomy, partial nephrectomy, and living-donor nephrectomy, with safety, and as an effective alternative to conventional laparoscopic procedures [37–39]. Various authors have also reported safe and effective robot-assisted laparoscopic adrenalectomy in humans [40–42]. Some authors even felt that the da Vinci system enables conventionally trained urologic surgeons to perform complex, minimally invasive procedures with ease and precision. The adrenal gland is small, vascular, and located in a difficult part of the body, and in such a situation the advantages of robotic assistance are tremendous. The biggest challenge, however, has been optimal positioning of the ports.

Robot-Assisted Pyeloplasty

Robot-assisted dismembered pyeloplasty was first reported in pigs, demonstrating the technical feasibility of the procedure with an acceptable morbidity

[43–45]. Different series of robotic pyeloplasty in humans have now been reported, with excellent outcomes. The most effective benefit is seen during spatulation and refashioning the flaps and during anastomosis [46–51]. In our experience of robot-assisted dismembered pyeloplasty for ureteropelvic junction obstruction (UPJ), we essentially followed the steps of open pyeloplasty. It allows clear inspection and preservation of crossing vessels, spatulation of the ureter, excision of the narrow portion of the UPJ, and fashioning of the pelvic flap. The ureteropelvic anastomosis is performed with our modified technique. The suture is prepared by tying two 4-0 monocryl sutures (dyed and undyed) to make a single suture with two needles. The anastomosis is started from the pelvic side to the ureter at the junction, then both sutures are carried upward to complete the anterior and posterior layers.

Female Urology

A variety of disorders in women can be repaired with robotic assistance, such as stress urinary incontinence, uterine prolapse, and pelvic floor weakness. Thus, there is a potential for reconstructive surgery for pelvic floor weakness with robotic assistance in women. Another interesting indication is myomectomy, in which an incision is essential if one wants to perform conventional surgery. In a limited experience at our center, robot-assisted hysterectomy, myomectomy, and pelvic floor repair were feasible, safe, and effective.

Male Infertility (Vasovasostomy and Vasoepididymostomy)

Robotic technology has been used for male reproductive microsurgery in a model of the vas deferens system using rat vasa deferentia. Full-thickness and mucosal anastomosis was performed using 10-0 bicurved nylon sutures. This drill was done by experienced and inexperienced microsurgeons, and both groups completed anastomoses with accuracy and enhanced comfort [52]. At our center, vasoepididymostomy and vasovasal anastomosis are being performed in patients for the reversal of primary and secondary infertility, respectively, with the assistance of the da Vinci robot. The EndoWrist black diamond microtip forceps was used to handling the 10-0 ethilon suture for anastomosis.

Conclusions

Laparoscopic robot-assisted urologic surgery is a fascinating technical development for the surgeon. The use of robotic assistance in performing and developing extirpative and reconstructive laparoscopic urologic surgical techniques has been evolving at a rapid pace. Over time it has become increasingly clear that anything that can be done by an open procedure can potentially be done with robotic assistance in laparoscopic urologic surgery. Hence, laparoscopic robotic urologic surgery is undoubtedly here to stay, although the challenge for the future is to continue to work to decide what procedures would be appropriate and most beneficial to patients with regard to safety, feasibility, efficacy, and efficiency, with improved outcomes, and also ergonomical to the surgeons. For example, at this time robotic radical prostatectomy is being used for the management of localized carcinoma of the prostate with obvious benefits in comparison to other techniques. Robot-assisted urologic surgery has also opened new vistas for telementoring and telerobotic surgery.

References

1. Hemal AK, Menon M (2002) Laparoscopy, robot, telesurgery and urology: future perspective. J Postgrad Med 48:39–41
2. Menon M, Hemal AK (2003) Laparoscopic surgery: where is it going? Prous Science: Timely Topics in Medicine, 10-10-2003, ttmed.com (epub)
3. Menon M, Shrivastava A, Sarle R, Hemal A, Tewari A. (2003) Vattikuti Institute Prostatectomy: a single-team experience of 100 cases. J Endourol 17:785–790
4. Menon M, Shrivastava A, Tewari A, Sarle R, Hemal A, Peabody JO, Vallancien G (2002) Laparoscopic and robot assisted radical prostatectomy: establishment of a structured program and preliminary analysis of outcomes. J Urol 168:945–949
5. Davies BL, Hibberd RD, Coptcoat MJ, Wickham JEA (1989) A surgeon robot prostatectomy—a laboratory evaluation. J Med Eng Technol 13:273–277
6. Satava RM (2002) Surgical robotics: a personal historical perspective. Surg Laparosc Endosc Percutan Tech 12:6–16
7. Walsh PC (1998) Anatomic radical prostatectomy: evolution of the surgical technique. J Urol 160:2418–2424
8. Guillonneau B, Vallancien G (2000) Laparoscopic radical prostatectomy: the Montsouris experience. J Urol 163:1643–1649
9. Schuessler WW, Schulam PG, Clayman RV, Kavoussi LR (1997) Laparoscopic radical prostatectomy: initial short-term experience. Urology 50:854–857
10. Abbou CC, Salomon L, Hoznek A, Antiphon P, Cicco A, Saint F, Alame W, Bello J, Chopin DK (2000) Laparoscopic radical prostatectomy: preliminary results. Urology 55:630–634
11. Gill IS, Zippe CD (2001) Laparoscopic radical prostatectomy with the Heilbronn technique: an analysis of the first 180 cases. Urol Clin North Am 28:423–436
12. Rassweiler J, Sentker L, Seemann O, Hatzinger M, Rumpelt HJ (2001) Laparoscopic radical prostatectomy with the Heilbronn technique: an analysis of the first 180 cases. J Urol 166:2101–2108
13. Tuerk I, Deger S, Winkelmann B, Loening SA (2001) Laparoscopic radical prostatectomy: technical aspects and experience with 125 cases. Eur Urol 40:46–52
14. Binder J, Kramer W (2001) Robotically-assisted laparoscopic radical prostatectomy. BJU Int 87:408–410
15. Abbou CC, Hoznek A, Salomon L, Olsson LE, Lobontiu A, Saint F, Cicco A, Antiphon P, Chopin D (2001) Laparoscopic radical prostatectomy with a remote controlled robot. J Urol 165(6 Pt 1):1964–1966
16. Rassweiler J, Frede T, Seemann O, Stock C, Sentker L (2001) Telesurgical laparoscopic radical prostatectomy. Initial experience. Eur Urol 40:75–83

17. Pasticier G, Rietbergen JB, Guillonneau B, Fromont G, Menon M, Vallancien G (2001) Robotically assisted laparoscopic radical prostatectomy: feasibility study in men. Eur Urol 40:70–74

18. Menon M, Shrivastava A, Sarle R, Hemal AK, Tewari A (2003) Vattikuti Institute Prostatectomy: a single team experience of 100 cases. J Endourol 17:785–790

19. Menon M (2003) Robotic radical retropubic prostatectomy. BJU Int 91:175–176

20. Ahlering TE, Skarecky D, Lee D, Clayman RV (2003) Successful transfer of open surgical skills to a laparoscopic environment using a robotic interface: initial experience with laparoscopic radical prostatectomy. J Urol 170:1738–1741

21. Bentas W, Wolfram M, Jones J, Brautigam R, Kramer W, Binder J (2003) Robotic technology and the translation of open radical prostatectomy to laparoscopy: the early Frankfurt experience with robotic radical prostatectomy and one year follow up. Eur Urol 44:175–181

22. Wolfram M, Brautigam R, Engl T, Bentas W, Heitkamp S, Ostwald M, Kramer W, Binder J, Blaheta R, Jonas D, Beecken WD (2003) Robotic-assisted laparoscopic radical prostatectomy: the Frankfurt technique. World J Urol 21:128–132

23. Tewari A, Peabody J, Sarle R, Balakrishnan G, Hemal A, Shrivastava A, Menon M (2002) Technique of da Vinci robot-assisted anatomic radical prostatectomy. Urology 60:569–572

24. Menon M, Tewari A, Peabody J, and members of the VIP Team (2003) Vattikuti Institute prostatectomy: technique. J Urol 169:2289–2292

25. Van Velthoven RF, Ahlering TE, Peltier A, Skarecky DW, Clayman RV (2003) Technique for laparoscopic running urethrovesical anastomosis: the single knot method. Urology 61:699–702

26. Menon M, Hemal AK, Tewari A, Shrivastava A, Bhandari A (2004) Technique of apical dissection of prostate and urethrovesical anastomosis in robotic radical prostatectomy. BJU Int. 2004 Apr; 93(6):715–719

27. Tewari A, Srivasatava A, Menon M, and members of the VIP Team (2003) A prospective comparison of radical retropubic and robot-assisted prostatectomy: experience in one institution. BJU Int 92:205–210

28. Menon M (2004) Laparoscopic radical prostatectomy: conventional and robotic. Lancet (in press)

29. Dalbagni G, Genega E, Hashibe M, Zhang ZF, Russo P, Herr H, Reuter V (2001) Cystectomy for bladder cancer: a contemporary series. J Urol 165:1111–1116

30. Gill IS, Kaouk JH, Meraney AM, Desai MM, Ulchaker JC, Klein EA, Savage SJ, Sung GT (2002) Laparoscopic radical cystectomy and continent orthotopic ileal neobladder performed completely intracorporeally: the initial experience. J Urol 168:13–18

31. Turk I, Deger S, Winkelmann B, Schonberger B, Loening SA (2001) Laparoscopic radical cystectomy with continent urinary diversion (rectal sigmoid pouch) performed completely intracorporeally: the initial 5 cases. J Urol 165:1863–1866

32. Hemal AK, Singh I, Kumar R (2004) Laparoscopic radical cystectomy and ileal conduit reconstruction: preliminary experience. J Endourol. 2003 Dec; 17(10):911–916

33. Menon M, Hemal AK, Tewari A, Shrivastava A, Shoma AM, El-Tabey NA, Shaaban A, Abol-Enein H, Ghoneim MA (2003) Nerve-sparing robot-assisted radical cystoprostatectomy and urinary diversion. BJU Int 92:232–236

34. Menon M, Hemal AK, Tewari A, Shrivastava A, Shoma AM, Abol-Enein H, Ghoneim MA (2004) Robot-assisted radical cystectomy and urinary diversion in female patients: technique with preservation of the uterus and vagina. J Am Coll Surg 198(3):386–393

35. Beecken WD, Wolfram M, Engl T, Bentas W, Probst M, Blaheta R, Oertl A, Jonas D, Binder J (2003) Robotic-assisted laparoscopic radical cystectomy and intra-abdominal formation of an orthotopic ileal neobladder. Eur Urol 44:337–339
36. Gill IS, Sung GT, Hsu TH, Meraney AM (2000) Robotic remote laparoscopic nephrectomy and adrenalectomy: the initial experience. J Urol 164:2082–2085
37. Talamini MA, Chapman S, Horgan S, Melvin WS (2003) A prospective analysis of 211 robotic-assisted surgical procedures. Surg Endosc Aug 15 (Epub ahead of print)
38. Horgan S, Vanuno D, Sileri P, Cicalese L, Benedetti E (2002) Robotic-assisted laparoscopic donor nephrectomy for kidney transplantation. Transplantation 73:1474–1479
39. Pinto PA, Fernando JK, Thomas WJ, Kavoussi LR (2004) Robot-assisted laparoscopic partial nephrectomy. J Endourol (in press)
40. Desai MM, Gill IS, Kaouk JH, Matin SF, Sung GT, Bravo EL (2002) Robotic-assisted laparoscopic adrenalectomy. Urology 60:1104–1107
41. Bentas W, Wolfram M, Brautigam R, Binder J (2002) Laparoscopic transperitoneal adrenalectomy using a remote-controlled robotic surgical system. J Endourol 16:373–376
42. Young A, Chapman WH III, Kim VB (2002) Robotic- assisted adrenalectomy for adrenal incidentaloma: case and review of the technique. Surg Laparosc Endosc Percutan Tech 12:126–130
43. Sung GT, Gill IS, Hsu TH (1999) Robotic assisted laparoscopic pyeloplasty: a pilot study. Urology 53:1099–1103
44. Guillonneau B, Rietbergen JB, Fromont G, Vallancien G (2003) Robotically assisted laparoscopic dismembered pyeloplasty: a chronic porcine study. Urology 61:1063–1066
45. Hubert J, Feuillu B, Mangin P, Lobontiu A, Artis M, Villemot JP (2003) Laparoscopic computer-assisted pyeloplasty: the results of experimental surgery in pigs. Br J Urol Int 92:437–440
46. Peschel R, Gettman M, Bartsch G (2003) Robotic- assisted laparoscopic pyeloplasty: initial clinical results. Eur Urol Suppl 2, No.1, pp 46
47. Hubert J, Feuillu B, Artis M (2003) Robotic remote laparoscopic treatment of UPJ syndrome: 18 cases. Eur Urol Suppl 2, No.1, pp 101
48. Gettman MT, Peschel R, Neururer R, Bartsch G (2002) A comparison of laparoscopic pyeloplasty performed with the da Vinci robotic system versus standard laparoscopic techniques: initial clinical results. Eur Urol 42:453–457; discussion, 457–458
49. Peter C (2002) Laparoscopic pyeloplasty: alternative techniques, robotics, and recent developments. Annual Meeting of the American Academy of Pediatrics, Boston, MA, USA, October 2002
50. Yohannes P, Burjonrappa SC (2003) Rapid communication: laparoscopic Anderson-Hynes dismembered pyeloplasty using the da Vinci robot: technical considerations. J Endourol 17:79–83
51. Bentas W, Wolfram M, Brautigam R, Probst M, Beecken WD, Jonas D, Binder J (2003) Da Vinci robot assisted Anderson-Hynes dismembered pyeloplasty: technique and 1 year follow-up. World J Urol 21:133–138
52. Schoor RA, Ross L, Niederberger C (2003) Robotic assisted microsurgical vassal reconstruction in a model system. World J Urol 21:48–49

Robotic Surgery Assisted by the ZEUS System

Masatoshi Eto and Seiji Naito

Summary. Urology has continuously embraced novel technologies, such as shockwave lithotripsy, lasers, and laparoscopy, that reduce patient morbidity yet maintain an excellent standard of care. To potentially increase the clinical applicability of laparoscopy, robots that enhance operative performance have recently been introduced for a variety of laparoscopic procedures, such as laparoscopic radical prostatectomy, pyeloplasty, and nephrectomy. Although the introduction of robotics has generated excitement, its benefits in large series of patients remain largely unknown. In this review, we mainly focus on one of the available robotic systems, the ZEUS system, and describe its features, including its advantages and limitations. We also review the emerging clinical applications of the ZEUS robotic system, including our recent cases of laparoscopic radical prostatectomy assisted by ZEUS, and the future potential of robotics in urology.

Keywords. Robotic surgery, ZEUS, Laparoscopy, Urology, Radical prostatectomy

Introduction

In the last 10 years, laparoscopy has revolutionized urology. However, many laparoscopic techniques (e.g., intracorporeal suturing) remain more difficult to perform than the corresponding tasks in open surgery. Furthermore, conventional laparoscopy imposes limitations on maneuverability (secondary to trocar positioning), vision (two-dimensional on flat screen), dexterity (secondary to long, awkward instruments), and tactile sensation when compared with open surgery. Therefore, robots that enhance operative performance may increase the applicability and precision of laparoscopy, yet decrease the learning curve of these minimally invasive tasks.

Department of Urology, Graduate School of Medical Sciences, Kyushu University, 3-1-1 Maidashi, Higashi-ku, Fukuoka 812-8582, Japan

Robots are increasingly utilized in urology, in part because of their favorable performance characteristics. Robots perform tasks quickly with excellent precision. Robots do not fatigue, regardless of time or environment, and can be more cost-effective than humans. The function of robots, however, remains heavily influenced by human factors. Indeed, industrial and medical robots function only as well as the software or operators controlling the devices. Recently, two performance-enhancing robots were introduced to increase the clinical applicability of laparoscopy [1–4]. One is the "da Vinci" system (Intuitive Surgical, Mountain View, CA, USA), and the other is the "ZEUS" system (Computer Motion, Goleta, CA, USA). In this manuscriptchapter, we focus on the ZEUS system and review the advantages and limitations of ZEUS and emerging clinical applications of ZEUS, including our recent cases of laparoscopic radical prostatectomy assisted by ZEUS.

Robotic System and Technical Factors

The ZEUS robot is a master–slave system consisting of two physically separated subsystems named "surgeon-side" and "patient-side" (Fig. 1a, b). The surgeon's subsystem has a console that takes the surgeon's input, and the patient's subsystem includes two robotic arms and the automated endoscope system for optimal positioning (AESOP). AESOP is designed to manipulate a laparoscope. The Food and Drug Administration (FDA) approved the use of AESOP in 1994. AESOP uses one mechanical arm with six degrees of freedom (DOFs) that is mounted to the operating table (Fig. 2a, b) [5–8]. AESOP is actively controlled by foot, hand, or voice commands. For increased safety, the laparoscope coupling mechanism disengages if more than 5 pounds of force is applied to the robotic arm during movement.

AESOP has been used for many laparoscopic procedures in multiple subspecialties. At Johns Hopkins University, Kavoussi et al. evaluated AESOP for urologic procedures, including ureterolysis, lymph node dissection, nephrectomy, and pyeloplasty [6]. The group found that AESOP maintained a steady image throughout surgery and eliminated the need for surgical assistants [6]. Kavoussi et al. performed a blinded study comparing laparoscopic manipulation by humans versus AESOP. With AESOP, the laparoscopic images were steadier and instrument collisions were decreased [7].

The main advantages of AESOP-assisted procedures are the excellent image quality and the steadiness of the operative view. With AESOP, surgeons depend less on human assistants while performing laparoscopy (Fig. 2c, d). AESOP has also made telementoring possible with laparoscopy [6, 9]. In this manner, an operator at a remote site (located even many kilometers away) can control the endoscope with AESOP for instructional purposes. For instance, researchers at the University of Innsbruck and Johns Hopkins University have previously reported the feasibility of laparoscopic telementoring for a procedure performed in Innsbruck, Austria, and telementored from Baltimore, Maryland, USA [9].

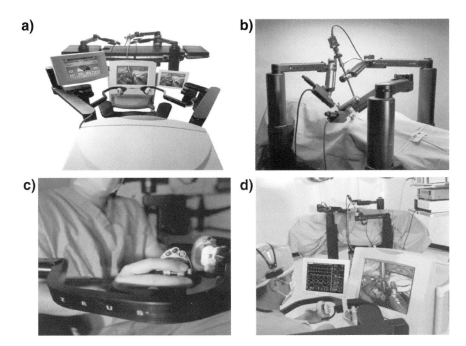

Fɪɢ. 1. ZEUS robotic systems. **a** The surgeon's robotic console. **b** Robotic arms on the patient's side. **c** The ergonomic handles of the recent version of ZEUS. **d** The new three-dimensional imaging system

AESOP is acquired with a relatively minimal capital investment, and the additional operative costs are minimal.

As with AESOP, the robotic arms are directly mounted to the operating table and are positioned through conventional trocars. A variety of surgical instruments can be connected to the robotic arms, so that the surgeon can activate the graspers, scissors, hook, and other instruments simply by manipulating the handles at the remote console. Standard ZEUS instruments have four DOFs, but newer articulating Microwrist instruments have five DOFs. All instruments are reusable and incorporate a durable pull-rod design. The surgeon sits in a comfortable chair in front of the video monitor, and the computer interface can eliminate the surgeon's resting tremor and be set to downscale the surgeon's hand movements over a range of 2:1 to 10:1. The recent version of ZEUS uses more ergonomic handles (Fig. 1c) and a Storz three-dimensional (3D) imaging system (Karl Storz Endoscopy, Tuttlingen, Germany) (Fig. 1d). The 3D imaging system is based on two separate right and left video cameras that visualize the operative field, a computer that merges and accelerates the broadcasted frames from the two video cameras, and a video monitor with an active matrix covering its surface. The surgeon wears glasses that have a clockwise polarizing filter as the right lens and a counterclockwise polarizing filter as the left lens, and that allow

a)   b)

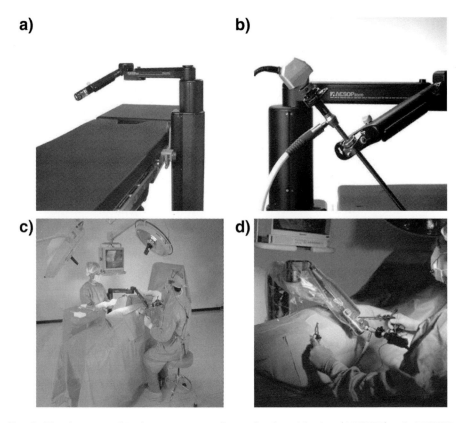

c)   d)

Fig. 2. The Automated endoscope system for optimal positioning (AESOP). **a,b** AESOP uses one mechanical arm with six degrees of freedom that is mounted on the operating table. **c,d** With AESOP, surgeons depend less on human assistants while performing laparoscopy

the left eye to see only images coming from the left camera while the right eye sees images from the right camera. This system causes a 3D image to be projected from the video monitor.

There are advantages and disadvantages of the ZEUS robotic system. Because the ZEUS components are mounted to the operating table, robotic adjustments relative to the patient are simplified. The open design of the ZEUS remote control unit also facilitates communication with scrubbed assistants. In addition, the availability of 3D imaging is advantageous for the system. Because new ZEUS instruments provide six DOFs, motion capabilities are better than those of standard laparoscopic instruments. Furthermore, many ZEUS instruments are already available, because designs are easily adapted from conventional laparoscopic instruments. On the other hand, the lack of an effective force-feedback feature is a disadvantage of ZEUS. Another disadvantage is the high initial capital investment for the robot, although ZEUS instruments are reusable.

Technical concerns have accompanied the introduction of master–slave systems. As with conventional laparoscopy, port placement is critical for successful robotic surgery. In general, ports should be arranged so the robot is best positioned for more challenging operative tasks (e.g., intracorporeal suturing). Optimal port placement for the ZEUS system can be affected by body habitus. For instance, if the distance between trocars is limited, performing ZEUS-assisted procedures can become more difficult. These factors may become more problematic in smaller patients. As the distance between trocars decreases, the exchange and alignment of instruments can become tedious. On the other hand, the effectiveness of robotic motion can also become restricted as the abdominal wall thickness increases. Thus, more frequent robotic positioning may be warranted to optimize robotic function. With ZEUS, however, since all robotic arms are independently mounted on the operating table, adjustments to accommodate body habitus can be more straightforward than with the da Vinci system. Robotic installation can be time consuming with telerobotic systems. Proper robotic installation also impacts performance of the laparoscopic procedures. Regardless of the robotic system, mechanical arms should be installed to maximize the range of motion of the robotic instruments.

Scrubbed assistants are critical to the success of telerobotic procedures. After assisting with trocar placement and robot positioning, scrubbed assistants exchange instruments on the robotic arms. Assistants also use conventional laparoscopic instruments for introduction and /removal of sutures, countertraction, suction, and assistance with hemostasis. The role of the assistant is especially important when non-robotic laparoscopic instruments are required (e.g., ultrasonic dissection, vascular stapling device, clip appliers, etc.). Most importantly, scrubbed assistants are immediately available if emergent laparotomy is required. Because of the distance separating the surgeon and the assistants, intraoperative communication can be impaired during telerobotics. In this regard, however, the open design of the ZEUS remote control unit may be advantageous to the periscope-type design of da Vinci.

As with conventional laparoscopy, a learning curve is present with telerobotic surgery. The robotic learning curve is thought, however, to be less steep than that of conventional laparoscopy. Since tactile feedback is essentially nonexistent with ZEUS and da Vinci, a learning curve exists for the performance of surgery preferentially with visual cues. In addition to suture breakage, lack of force feedback can also contribute to inadvertent tissue damage. A learning curve is also present when the magnified three-dimensional imaging systems are used, especially for surgeons accustomed to performing conventional laparoscopy on a standard video monitor [10]. The learning curve can be minimized by performing telerobotic procedures in familiar surroundings with the same team [11]. In the event the robot should fail, the surgeon should also have experience with intracorporeal suturing. In that case, the surgeon could finish with laparoscopy instead of converting to open surgery. Other groups, however, have evaluated the impact of using ZEUS for instructing medical students, surgical residents, and surgeons in advanced laparoscopic techniques [12–14]. In summary, these studies showed that, whereas robotic assistance conferred little or no advantage on the performance of simple tasks, suturing or other more complex tasks were accomplished with greater speed and precision when performed with ZEUS, regardless of the prior level of training of each surgeon. These data suggest that robotic assistance might facilitate the learning and performance of complex laparoscopic operations.

Laparoscopic Applications of ZEUS

Renal and Adrenal

Robots have previously been utilized experimentally and clinically for upper urinary tract applications [13, 15, 16]. Gill et al. first reported the feasibility of laparoscopic telerobotic nephrectomy and adrenalectomy in the animal model using the ZEUS robot [13]. In that study, telerobotic procedures were compared with standard techniques for laparoscopic nephrectomy, and adrena-lectomy was performed in five farm pigs. The operative times were slower with robotics, but the adequacy of dissection and blood loss were equivalent [13]. Sung and Gill performed a head-to-head comparison of the da Vinci robotic system with the ZEUS robotic system for laparoscopic nephrectomy, adrenalectomy, and pyeloplasty [15]. Although feasibility was proven with each system, the operative times and learning curve were more favorable with da Vinci. Furthermore, the researchers concluded that operative motions were more intuitive with da Vinci [15]. The first telerobotic nephrectomy in humans was reported by Guillonneau et al. using the ZEUS robot [16]. All steps of telerobotic nephrectomy were successfully performed with an operative time of 200 min and an estimated blood loss of less than 100 ml [16]. To date, a larger experience with telerobotics for nephrectomy has not been reported. Although the feasibility of robotic adrenalectomy has also been reported with da Vinci in humans [17, 18], so far there is no report of robotic adrenalectomy with ZEUS.

Telerobotic laparoscopic pyeloplasty has also been performed clinically and in the animal model. The feasibility of laparoscopic pyeloplasty was first reported by Sung et al. using female farm pigs randomized to undergo surgery with or without the ZEUS robot [19]. When robotic and non-robotic procedures were compared, the differences in operative time, suturing time, and number of suture-bites per ureter were not significant [19]. In humans, robotic-assisted laparoscopic pyeloplasty with both the da Vinci and the ZEUS robotic systems has been described [20, 21]. In addition, when patients undergoing da Vinci-assisted laparoscopic Fengerplasty or Anderson–Hynes pyeloplasty were compared with patients undergoing the corresponding procedures without the robot, the da Vinci-assisted procedures were associated with shorter operative times and decreased suturing times [22]. To date, however, a large experience with ZEUS-assisted pyeloplasties has not been reported.

Prostate

Given the difficulty of laparoscopic radical prostatectomy (LRP) and the incidence of prostate cancer, telerobotics has generated significant clinical interest among urologists. Guillonneau et al. [23] performed robotic-assisted, laparoscopic pelvic lymph-node dissection in 10 consecutive patients with T3M0 prostatic carcinoma and compared the operative, postoperative, and pathological parameters with the results from their last 10 patients undergoing conventional laparoscopic pelvic lymph-node dissection for similar indications by the same operator. The authors reported no specific intraoperative or postoperative complications in the robotic group. The mean operating time for the robotic group was 125 ± 57 min (range, 75 to 215), significantly longer than that with conventional laparoscopic experience ($p < 0.01$). As for radical prostatectomy, Tewari and Menon recently reported excellent results for 250 cases of a robot-assisted radical prostatectomy using the da Vinci system [24]. The mean operating time for their robot-assisted radical prostatectomy was 2.5 h, and the average blood loss was 150 ml. Thus, the use of robot-assisted radical prostatectomy with the da Vinci system is now spreading. However, so far there has been no report on a robot-assisted radical prostatectomy using the ZEUS system. We recently performed an LRP assisted by the ZEUS robotic system. The ZEUS system was utilized only for vesicourethral anastomosis, one of the most difficult procedures to perform during LRP. The vesicourethral anastomosis using the ZEUS system, however, required 100 min, which was not shorter than our average anastomosis time without ZEUS (data not shown). Since this is our first case with ZEUS, we believe that we can shorten the operation time as we increase our experience with the ZEUS system. The urethral catheter was removed 7 days after the operation without any postoperative complications. In our case, we utilized the ZEUS system only for vesicourethral anastomosis, whereas Tewari and Menon used the da Vinci system for all LRP procedures. We therefore cannot directly compare the two results. However, one of the disadvantages of the current robotic systems is lack of an effective force-feedback feature. The lack of tactile feedback can sometimes cause inadvertent tissue damage. Taken together, since the conversion to the ZEUS system from conventional laparoscopic surgery is easier than that to the da Vinci system, the utilization of the ZEUS system only for vesicourethral anastomosis in LRP may become an alternative method to optimize the merit of the ZEUS system. After performing more LRP procedures using the ZEUS system, we will thus be able to better answer the question of which robotic system is most suitable for LRP.

Bladder

Although the first da Vinci-assisted laparoscopic cystectomy and ileal neoblad-der has been performed (personal communication, J. Binder, Frankfurt, Germany, 2002) based on the clinical experience with da Vinci-assisted LRP, so far there is no report of ZEUS-assisted laparoscopic cystectomy. In the animal model, Cho et al. have compared the performance of extravesical ureteral re-implantations with and without the ZEUS robotic system [25]. Procedures per-formed with the ZEUS robotic system required significantly more operative time, but all reimplantations were immediately water-tight, and the suturing characteristics were comparable between treatment groups. For robotic applica-tions involving the lower urinary tract, additional clinical data are not available at this time.

Current Limitations and Future Perspectives

One of the major technical criticisms of robotic systems is that they are associ-ated with a lack of tactile feedback from the operating instruments, which is only in part compensated for by the 3D visual feedback. This may be a temporary drawback, as technology evolves rapidly and significant research efforts are focusing on the issue of providing tactile feedback to robotic systems. Recently, a group of scientists in Spain has developed a robotic finger with a sense of touch. This robotic finger can feel the weight of what it is pushing and adjust the energy it uses accordingly [26]. This report is promising and suggests that in the fore-seeable future, technologic advances may overcome, at least in part, the lack of tactile sensation characteristic of current robotic systems.

The feasibility and safety of robotic laparoscopy have been reported in clini-cal and experimental studies. Experiences in different centers, both clinically and experimentally, show that the use of the ZEUS system does not result in specific complications and achieves outcomes similar to those of standard laparoscopic procedures. It is a common finding, however, that the use of ZEUS increases the operative time. Furthermore, all clinical studies performed so far have failed to provide any evidence of specific patient benefits in general surgical procedures. Although the lack of verifiable clinical benefits may be frustrating, the demon-stration of the feasibility and safety of using the ZEUS system for several sur-gical procedures should be seen as an encouraging starting point. The merging of robotics with computer technologies and virtual reality may also impact future generations of robots.

Telecommunication may also impact robotics. With current technology, tele-mentoring is an accepted discipline in laparoscopic surgery. The most important limitation on the performance of robotic-assisted procedures across long dis-tances was considered to be the reliability (or quality of service) of telecommu-nication lines and the issue of latency (the delay from the time when the hand motion is initiated by the surgeon until the manipulator actually moves and the image is shown on the surgeon's monitor). Due to the latency factor, it was believed that the feasible distance for remote surgery was no more than a few hundred miles over terrestrial telecommunications [27]. With current telecommunications using dedicated asynchronous transfer mode (ATM) fibers, however, telerobotic surgery has been reported for human laparoscopic cholecystectomy between New York and Strasbourg, France [28]. The ZEUS system was used in all steps of that project. The mean time delay over transoceanic distances was 155 msec with the ATM fibers. This extremely short delay allowed the safe performance of remote laparoscopic cholecystectomy. With telecommunication and computing advances, the ease of telesurgery may increase, but clinical necessity remains unproven. The licensure and liability issues of telesurgery must also be resolved [29]. Cost is also a drawback at the moment. In spite of these limitations, however, the potential benefits of remote surgery are multiple. Many abdominal operations can indeed be performed laparoscopically now, but complex procedures are still in the hands of a limited number of experts. Remote robotic assistance may provide useful help to inexperienced surgeons in the early phase of the learning curve. Furthermore, patients will be able to receive the type of treatment best suited to their conditions, ideally in any part of the world. We will have to find out the best way to optimize the merit of the ZEUS system.

References

1. Hoznek A, Zaki SK, Samadi DB, Salomon L, Lobontiu A, Lang P, Abbou CC (2002) Robotic assisted kidney transplantation: an initial experience. J Urol 167:1604–1606
2. Darzi A, Mackay S (2002) Recent advances in minimal access surgery. BMJ 324:31–34
3. Felger JE, Nifong LW, Chitwood WR (2001) Robotic cardiac valve surgery: transcending the technologic crevasse!. Curr Opin Cardiol 16:146–151
4. Hashizume M, Konishi K, Tsutsumi N (2002) A new era of robotic surgery assisted by a computer-enhanced surgical system. Surgery 131:S330–S333
5. Cadeddu JA, Stoianovici D, Kavoussi LR (1997) Robotics in urologic surgery. Urology 49:501–506
6. Kavoussi LR, Moore RG, Partin AW, Bender JS, Zenilman ME, Satava RM (1994) Telerobotic assisted laparoscopic surgery: initial laboratory and clinical experience. Urology 44:15–19
7. Kavoussi LR, Moore RG, Adams JB, Partin AW (1995) Comparison of robotic versus human laparoscopic camera control. J Urol 154:2134–2136
8. Partin AW, Adams JB, Moore RG, Kavoussi LR (1995) Complete robot-assisted laparoscopic urologic surgery: a preliminary report. J Am Coll Surg 181:552–557
9. Janetschek G, Bartsch G, Kavoussi LR (1998) Transcontinental interactive laparoscopic telesurgery between the United States and Europe. J Urol 160:1413
10. Rassweiler J, Binder J, Frede T (2001) Robotic and telesurgery: will they change our future?. Curr Opin Urol 11:309–320
11. Abbou CC, Hoznek A, Salomon L, Olsson LE, Lobontiu A, Saint AF, Cicco A, Antiphon P, Chopin D (2001) Laparoscopic radical prostatectomy with remote controlled robot. J Urol 165:1964–1966

12. Garcia-Ruiz A, Ganger M, Miller JH, Steiner CP, Hahn JF (1998) Manual vs roboti-cally assisted laparoscopic surgery in the performance of basic manipulation and suturing tasks. Arch Surg 133:957–961
13. Gill IS, Sung GT, Hsu TH, Meraney AM (2000) Robotic remote laparoscopic nephrec-tomy and adrenalectomy: the initial experience. J Urol 164:2082–2085
14. Nio D, Bemelman A, Kuenzler R, den Bore K, Gouma DJ, van Gulik TM (2001) Effi-ciency of manual versus robotic (ZEUS) assisted laparoscopic surgery in the per-formance of standardized tasks: a random trial. Surg Endosc 15:S150
15. Sung GT, Gill IS (2001) Robotic laparoscopic surgery: a comparison of the da Vinci and Zeus ZEUS systems. Urology 58:893–898
16. Guillonneau B, Jayet C, Tewari A, Vallancien G (2001) Robot assisted laparoscopic nephrectomy. J Urol 166:200–201
17. Young JA, Chapman, 3rd WH III, Kim VB, Albrecht RJ, Ng PC, Nifong LW, Chitwood, WR Jr WR (2002) Robotic-assisted adrenalectomy for adrenal inciden-taloma: case and review of the technique. Surg Laparosc Endosc Percutan Tech 12:126–130
18. Bentas W, Wolfram M, Brautigam R, Binder J (2002) Laparoscopic transperitoneal adrenalectomy using a remote controlled robotic surgical system. J Endourol 16:373–376
19. Sung GT, Gill IS, Hsu TH (1999) Robotic-assisted laparoscopic pyeloplasty: a pilot study. Urology 53:1099–1103
20. Graham RW, Graham SD, Bokinsky GB (2001) Urological upper tract surgery with the da Vinci robotic system, pyeloplasty. J Urol 165(SupplSuppl):V74
21. Guilloneau B, Jayet C, Cappele O, Vallancien G (2001) Robotic-assisted laparoscopic pyeloplasty. J Urol 165(SupplSuppl):V75
22. Gettman MT, Peschel R, Neururer R, Bartsch G (2002) Laparoscopic pyeloplasty: comparison of procedures performed with the da Vinci robotic system versus stan-dard techniques. Eur Urol 42:453–458
23. Guilloneau B, Cappele O, Martinez JB, Navarra S, Vallancien G (2001) Robotic assisted laparoscopic pelvic lymph node dissection in humans. J Urol 165:1078–1081
24. Tewari A, Menon M (2003) Vattikuti Institute prostatectomy: surgical technique and current results. Curr Urol Rep 4:119–123
25. Cho WY, Sung GT, Meraney AM, Gill IS (2001) Remote robotic laparoscopic extravesical ureteral reimplantation with ureteral advancement technique. J Urol 165(Suppl):V640
26. Otero TF, Cortes MT (2003) Artificial muscles with tactile sensitivity. Adv Mater Weinheim 15:279–282
27. Mack MJ (2001) Minimally invasive and robotic surgery. JAMA 285:568–572
28. Marescaux J, Leroy J, Gagner M, Rubino F, Mutter D, Vix M, Butner SE, Smith MK (2001) Transatlantic robot-assisted telesurgery. Nature 413:379–380
29. Stanberry B (2000) Telemedicine: barriers and opportunities in the 21st century. J Int Med 247:615–628

Telesurgery: Remote Monitoring and Assistance During Laparoscopy

Takeshi Inagaki, Sam B. Bhayani, and Louis R. Kavoussi

Summary. Laparoscopic surgery is the most commonly practiced and accepted form of minimally invasive surgery. Laparoscopic surgery in urology has, in many instances, become the standard of care. However, laparoscopy is associated with a steep learning curve because of its complexity and difficulty. This learning curve causes long operative times and potentially increases operative complications. Interestingly, to date there are no formal credentialing guidelines. Telesurgery has become feasible with the advent of recent Internet and robotic technology. This new technology has applicability within urology, as it enables an expert laparoscopic surgeon to mentor an inexperienced surgeon from a remote location. In this article, we review the background to current telesurgical research and describe experiences, with emphasis on the current status of this technology within urology. Telesurgery is feasible and may play a major role within urology. Although the utility of this technology is apparent, especially within minimally invasive approaches, barriers such as technical limitations and legal implications may hinder its progress and eventual acceptance. Urologists standing at the beginning of the twenty-first century should be cognizant of the eventual implementation of this technology.

Keywords. Laparoscopy, Telesurgery, Telementoring, Robot

Introduction

During the past 20 years, minimally invasive surgery has influenced the techniques used in every specialty of surgery. Laparoscopic surgery has been the most visible aspect of minimally invasive surgery. Laparoscopy not only has supplanted conventional procedures, but also has stimulated surgeons to reevaluate conventional approaches with regard to perioperative parameters such as post-

The James Buchanan Brady Urological Institute, The Johns Hopkins Medical Institutions, 600 North Wolfe Street, Suite 161, Jefferson Street Bldg, Baltimore, MD 21287-8915, USA

49

operative pain, cosmesis, recovery, and length of hospital stay. As in general surgery and gynecology, laparoscopic surgery has a great role in the realm of urologic surgery. The initial emphasis was on ablative procedures [1–3]. Ratner and his coworkers reported the first laparoscopic donor nephrectomy in 1995. This has become a standard operation [4]. As urologists became more skilled, the most challenging aspect of laparoscopy became reconstructive surgery. With the development of suturing and intracorporeal knot tying, many reconstructive procedures were successfully completed laparoscopically [5]. Additionally, laparoscopic surgery began to expand into such technically advanced surgeries as radical cystectomy [6, 7] and radical prostatectomy [8].

Although laparoscopy has moved into the mainstream of urologic surgery, one major drawback has emerged. The ability of surgeons to perform laparoscopic surgery improves significantly as they gain experience with the procedure. This is the so-called learning curve, and the drawback is that learning curve for most surgeons is still steep because of complexity and technical difficulties, in comparison with the learning process in open surgery. Furthermore, complications may be more common during a surgeon's initial experience with laparoscopy [9].

Telemedicine is a rapidly developing field that takes advantage of the information highway to provide physicians and patients with global access to health care [10]. In laparoscopic surgery, all members of the surgical staff, including the primary surgeon, assistant surgeon, and operation room staff, watch the same laparoscopic images. Therefore, transferring of laparoscopic images readily influences education and assistance in laparoscopic surgery. In that context, laparoscopic surgery is the most appropriate surgery that adopts telesurgical technology. Telesurgery, a subcategory of telemedicine, would enable a laparoscopic surgeon to educate a less experienced surgeon from a remote place [11]. In this article, we review the background of current telesurgical research and describe clinical experiences.

Background

Definitions of Terms

Teleproctoring: Teleproctoring is the monitoring and evaluation of surgical trainees from a distance. In its most simple form, teleproctoring can provide one-way communication from the local operating room to the remote specialist workstation. The use of modern telecommunications in proctoring for the purpose of granting of hospital privileges, specialty board credentialing, and training has the potential to make a significant impact. Its enables the expanded use of real-time skill assessment and technique surveillance [12].

Teleconsultation: Teleconsultation involves transmission of still or video images for review by a remote specialist, who then communicate his or her opinions to the local surgeon [13].

Telementoring: Telementoring involves the remote real-time guidance of a treatment or a surgical procedure where the local doctor has no or limited experience [13]. This interaction requires two-way communication by video and audio, which must occur simultaneously between the local and the remote site. Furthermore, it is mandatory that the time lag of this communication be as short as possible.

Robotic surgery: The Robot Institute of the USA defines a robot as "a programmable multifunctional manipulator designed to move materials, parts, tools, or specialized devices through variable programmed motions for the performance of a variety of tasks" [14]. The first robots introduced into clinical surgical procedures were controlled directly by the surgeon at the operating room table [15, 16]. More recently, robotic surgery has involved active control of surgical instruments, such as graspers, electrocautery, scissors, etc., by a surgeon located at a remote site [17–20].

Telepresence surgery: The success of telerobotic surgery has spurred interest in telepresence surgery. Telepresence surgery is defined as an operation controlled by a remote surgeon via telerobotic technology [21, 22].

Other technical terms used in telesurgery, especially in data transmission, are listed briefly in Table 1.

Types of Communication Links

Telesurgery is dependent on reliable data transmission between the primary operating room and the remote site. Conventional telephone and modem, Ethernet, ISDN, ADSL, and ATM are currently used for transmission of information (Table 2) [23, 24]. In telesurgery, time delay in the transmission of surgical information is a major problem. Currently, ISDN is the most frequently used mode of transmission, and three or four ISDN lines are generally used for telesurgical transmission [25]. Janetschek et al. reported that the time delay for telementoring between Innsbruck in Austria and Baltimore in the United States using three ISDN lines was 1 second, which did not present a problem for transcontinental telementoring [26]. However, three ISDN lines provide only 384 kbps, and the sharpness of the transmitted image is limited. ATM provides high-speed packet switching data services, and a mean time delay of 155 ms over a transoceanic distance was reported [21]. Technical surveys of network architectures for teleradiology suggest that ATM is the most reliable high-speed switching network available for this application [27].

Currently Available Robotic Systems

Telesurgery is usually carried out by using various surgical robots.

TABLE 1. Definition of technical terms used in telesurgery

Term	Definition
ATM	Asynchronous transfer mode: a high-speed and high-quality terrestrial fiberoptic network
Bandwidth	The amount of data that can be transmitted over a line or channel in a fixed amount of time. A higher bandwidth results in higher information-carrying capacity
Broadband	A high-speed, high-capacity transmission channel
Cable modem	Digital modem that supports Internet access using the coaxial cable provided by cable television providers. Bandwidth is approximately 2 Mbps
DICOM	Digital imaging and communication in medicine
DSL	Digital subscriber lines: sophisticated modulation schemes that pack large amounts of data onto copper telephone wires. Now available to consumers, these systems provide high-bandwidth connections to the Internet (as high as 32 Mbps)
Duplex	Transmission of data between parties simultaneously in both directions
Encryption	Translation of data into code for security purposes. To read encrypted data, the recipient must have access to a key that enables decryption
Force-feedback	Transmission of force information from a remote instrument back to the operator in an attempt to simulate tactile sensation
Frame rate	A measure of how information is used to store and display motion video. Each frame is a still image, and the frame rate is described as frames per second (fps)
ISDN	Integrated services digital network: an international standard for transmitting data over digital telephone lines. Supports transfer rates in increments of 64 Kbps
Time lag	Time delay for an instruction to be encoded on a local machine, propagated over a transmission line to a remote machine, decoded, and executed

TABLE 2. Types of communication links and their data transfer speed

Network	Typical speeds (kbps)
Local area network	
Ethernet	10,000
Fast ethernet	100,000
Wide area networking	
Telephone and modem	56
ISDN	64–128
Broadband ISDN	384
Broadband ISDN	631
ADSL	512–2,000
ATM	25,000–155,000

Kbps, kilobits per second; ISDN, integrated services digital network; ADSL, asynchronous digital subscriber line; ATM, asynchronous transfer mode

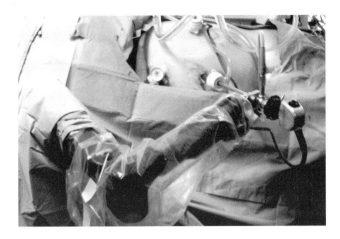

Fɪɢ. 1. AESOP (automated endoscopic system for optimal positioning) camera holder enables a single surgeon to perform a laparoscopic procedure

AESOP

AESOP (automated endoscopic system for optimal positioning) was initially approved by the US Food and Drug Administration (FDA) for clinical use in 1994. AESOP's arm was modified to hold a laparoscope. Initially AESOP was attached to the operating table and controlled manually or remotely with a foot switch or hand control [27, 28]. More recently AESOP may be controlled by voice activation (Fig. 1) [29].

PAKY

PAKY (percutaneous access to the kidney) is a radiolucent, sterilizable needle driver located at the terminal end of the robot arm. The needle driver utilizes an axial-loaded rotational-to-translational friction transmission principle to grasp, stabilize, and advance an 18-gauge access needle into the kidney percutaneously. Needle insertion is driven by a variable-speed, battery-powered DC motor [30].

Da Vinci

The first telerobotic surgery system was developed by Green and colleagues at the Stanford Research Institute (SRI International, California, USA) in 1992 [31]. This system was then developed commercially as the MOMA telesurgery system (Intuitive Surgical, California, USA), and was later improved and renamed the da Vinci telesurgery system 17]. The da Vinci system now uses

EndoWrist technology, giving the arm seven degrees of freedom in its articulated movement, and has two cameras to allow a three-dimensional view to be presented through a specialized binocular arrangement [18, 19].

ZEUS

The ZEUS system (Computer Motion, California, USA) is similar in design to the da Vinci system. It has robotic arms on the patient side that attach directly to the operating table, and the surgical site is viewed on the screen by the theater staff. The ZEUS system uses a voice-controlled AESOP robotic arm (Computer Motion) to hold a camera and has a range of laparoscopic instruments that attach to the other two arms [18, 20].

Progress to Date

In the realm of pathology and radiology, teleconsultation for pathological diagnosis and radiological diagnosis has been refined in the last decade. One of the first reports of real-time teleconsultation was published by Kyser and Drlicek in 1992 [32]. They transferred histopathological images of intraoperative sections by use of normal telephone lines between two departments of pathology. It was reported that the transfer of an image lasted for 1.4 to 2 min, and the expert discussion was finished 3 min after the transfer of the last image. Using the Internet as a telecommunication pathway for static images is a low-cost, widely available option [33, 34]. Recently, dynamic telepathology has used remote-controlled microscope systems with high-throughput online image-transport channels [35]. This method has the advantage of entire slide access and prevent errors from preselected microscopical frames. On the other hand, internet technology has enabled computed tomographic (CT) images and magnetic resonance images (MRI) to be downloaded from a centralized server and displayed at a remote hospital or a radiologist's home [36–38]. Tachakra et al. reported that teleradiological consultation is effective to prevent patients from being transferred unnecessarily [39].

In general surgery, Chinnock reported that since virtual reality systems have become digitally based, they have become capable of being put on line for tele-training, consulting, and even surgery [40]. In addition, surgical teleproctoring during laparoscopic surgery was reported by Hiatt and his coworkers [41]. In 1997, Rosser telementored laparoscopic colectomies performed by inexperienced surgeons [42]. This area has been of particular interest to military and National Aeronautics and Space Administration (NASA) surgeons who face the challenges of emergency procedures in remote locations, aboard ships at sea, or in space [43–45]. Cubano et al. reported five laparoscopic hernia repairs performed successfully abroad the USS Abraham Lincoln Aircraft Carrier Battle group under remote telementoring guidance [43]. In Japan, the telecommunication center was established at Osaka and has been operational since 1997 using six ISDN channels. The network, composed of five remote hospitals, aimed to teleeducate young surgeons in constituent hospitals, and it was applied not only to teleeducation in routine endoscopic surgery, but also to telementoring in advanced operations [46].

Urological Telementoring

Trials have been reported of the use of telementoring in urological procedures. In 1994, Kavoussi and coworkers reported that cholecystectomy, bladder suspension, and valix ligation were successfully performed using the AESOP robotic arm controlled by an experienced surgeon at a remote site (Fig. 2) [47]. Since then, Kavoussi's group has tried to extend the distance between the remote site and the primary operating site. The remote-site surgeon, located in a control room over 1000 feet away from the operating room, supervised an inexperienced surgeon. Data were transferred via fiberoptic and copper wire links. The remote surgeon was capable of simultaneously viewing internal and external images of the primary operating room and could control the laparoscope and draw an overlay video sketch on the video image generated by the internal camera [48, 49]. This overlay sketch appeared on the internal operative video monitor at the primary site. They developed a system that connected a central site (Johns Hopkins Hospital) and an operating site (the Bayview Campus of the Johns Hopkins Medical Institute, approximately 3.5 miles apart) via a single T1 (1.54 Mbs) point-to-point communication link. The system provided a real-time video display from either the laparoscope or an externally mounted camera located in the operating room, full duplex audio, telestration over live video, control of a robotic arm that manipulated the laparoscope, and access to electrocautery for tissue cutting or hemostasis [50].

The group at Johns Hopkins subsequently attempted telementoring surgery over international and intercontinental distances. The telementoring remote site in Baltimore (USA) was connected to operating sites in Innsbruck (Austria),

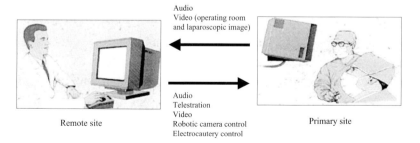

Audio
Video (operating room
and laparoscopic image)

Audio
Telestration
Video
Robotic camera control
Electrocautery control

Remote site

Primary site

FIG. 2. The illustrated telementoring system developed at the Johns Hopkins School of Medicine

Bangkok (Thailand), Singapore, Rome (Italy), and Munich (Germany) [27, 51–56]. The first transcontinental telementoring involved a laparoscopic adrenalectomy performed between Baltimore and Innsbruck. Recently, a laparoscopic bilateral varicocelectomy and a percutaneous renal access for a percutaneous nephrolithotripsy were performed with telementoring assistance between Baltimore and São Paulo and Recife (Brazil) [57]. Four ISDN lines, each line carrying 128 kbps, were used for data transfer between the primary operating site and the remote site. AESOP was applied for laparoscopic varicocelectomy, and PAKY was used for percutaneous renal access. The remote surgeon was capable of making notes and drawings over the full-motion video monitor. Furthermore, the two surgical robots, AESOP and PAKY, were controlled by the remote surgeon. Both surgeries were successfully completed. In 2003, Ushiyama and coworkers reported the performance of laparoscopic adrenalectomy under telementoring guidance. They used a fiberoptic cable for data transfer between the primary site and the remote site about 100 m away [25]. Telementoring trials at the Johns Hopkins Medical Institute are summarized in Table 3.

Robotic Surgery in Urology

Robots designed for surgery have three potential advantages over humans: three-dimensional spatial accuracy, reliability, and the capability of achieving much greater precision. Surgical robots were initially used in neurosurgery and orthopedics. Surgical robots were used for stereotactic framing in neurosurgery [15], and a robot was used to cut and ream bones with great precision for the fitting of joint prostheses or for replacing ligaments [16]. In urology, robotic systems have been developed to assist with intraoperative percutaneous renal access [58], transperineal prostate biopsy [59], radioactive seed delivery into the prostate [60], and transurethral resection of the prostate [61]. Kavoussi and coworkers compared the control of the endoscope by AESOP with control by the assistant, and they reported the usefulness of this robotic camera control system [62].

Advancement of the technology enabled surgeons to control robots from remote sites. The next logical step will be to implement active robotic instruments, such as the grasper, scissors, cautery, and so on, that can be controlled remotely. This area has rapidly advanced, and new robot systems have been developed, such as ZEUS and da Vinci [18–20]. These robots function as a master-slave system, in which the device transmits the movement of the hand of the surgeon to the surgical instrument by remote manipulation.

Problems in Telesurgery

Transferring speed, image quality, and the amount of transferable data may be considered technical problems. On the other hand, the protection of personal information and privacy and malpractice liability are considered legal problems.

TABLE 3. Telementoring trials in Johns Hopkins University

Reference	System	Transfer	Procedures	Success rate (mentoring)	Comments
Kavoussi 1994 [47]	Audiovisual AESOP	Fiber optic cable	3 laparoscopic surgeries	3/3	Initial trial
Schulan 1997 [50]	Audiovisual AESOP, telestrator	T1 line	7 laparoscopic surgeries	7/7	Telementored 5 km away
Moore 1996 [48]	Audiovisual AESOP, telestrator	Fiber optic cable	23 laparoscopic surgeries (14 advanced, 9 basic)	22/23	One improper positioning of robotic arm
Cheriff 1996 [49]	Audiovisual AESOP, telestrator	Fiber optic cable	6 laparoscopic surgeries (6 complex cases)	6/6	Telementored 300 m away
Lee 1998 [52]	Audiovisual AESOP, telestrator	3 ISDN lines	3 laparoscopic surgeries	3/3	Between USA and Austria, Thailand
Janetshek 1998 [26]	Audiovisual AESOP, telestrator	3 ISDN lines	Laparoscopic adrenalectomy	1/1	Between USA and Austria
Lee 2000 [53]	Audiovisual AESOP, telestrator	3 ISDN lines	2 laparoscopic surgeries	2/2	Between USA and Singapore
Bove 2003 [56]	AESOP, PAKY Audiovisual Telestrator	3 or 4 ISDN lines	14 laparoscopic surgeries 3 percutaneous approaches	10/17	Between USA and Italy
Rodrigues 2003 [57]	AESOP, PAKY Audiovisual Telestrator	3 or 4 ISDN lines	1 laparoscopic surgery 1 percutaneous approach	2/2	Between USA and Brazil

Conventional telephones and modems, Ethernet, ISDN, ADSL, and ATM are currently used for the transmission of information. ISDN is the most popular, and three or four ISDN lines are generally used for telesurgical transmission [56]. During 1999, new broad-band technologies, such as cable modems and digital subscriber lines (DSL), became widely available. These communication technologies should accelerate the development of telesurgical systems by providing affordable, high-speed, high-bandwidth Internet access [13]. Average cable modem connections operate at 1.5 to 2 Mbps, a bandwidth almost 36 times greater than standard 56 Kbps analog modems. These new technologies could facilitate telesurgical mentoring at remote medical sites not directly hardwired to the Internet backbone. ATM provides high-speed packet-switching data services and high quality of images with transmission rates of 155 Mbits/s. Furthermore, ATM provides high-level security services, and technical surveys of network architectures for teleradiology suggest that ATM is the most reliable high-speed switching network available for this application [63].

Patient privacy issues have become more complex, as a great proportion of medical records are stored and transmitted in electronic form [64]. In telesurgery, if patient information is leaked or patient privacy is infringed, the medical institution and/or the telecommunications industry may be unduly exposed to legal ramifications. In order to perform telesurgery privately, the encryption of information and data authentication must be introduced, and advanced security technology is required in telesurgical communication [65]. Malpractice liability in telesurgery is a complex topic. Although the legal issues are not yet defined, the potential medical benefits are enormous. The medical and legal community will work together to develop the ethical and medicolegal framework to perform telesurgery safely.

References

1. Schuessler WW, Vancaillie TG, Reich H, Griffith DP (1991) Transperitoneal endosurgical lymphadenectomy in patients with localized prostate cancer. J Urol 145:988–991
2. Clayman RV, Kavoussi LR, Soper NJ, Dierks SM, Merety KS, Darcy MD, Long SR, Roemer FD, Pingleton ED, Thomson PG (1991) Laparoscopic nephrectomy. N Engl J Med 324:1370–1371
3. Sanchez-de-Badajoz E, Diaz-Ramirez F, Vara-Thorbeck C (1990) Endoscopic varicocelectomy. J Endourol 4:371–374
4. Ratner LE, Ciseck LJ, Moore RG, Cigarroa FG, Kaufman HS, Kavoussi LR (1995) Laparoscopic live donor nephrectomy. Transplantation 60:1047–1049
5. Kaouk JH, Gill IS (2003) Laparoscopic reconstructive urology. J Urol 170:1070–1075
6. Raboy A, Ferzli G, Albert P (1997) Initial experience with extraperitoneal endoscopic radical retropubic prostatectomy. Urology 50:849–853
7. Schuessler W, Schulam P, Clayman R, Kavoussi L (1997) Laparoscopic radical prostatectomy: initial short-term experience. Urology 50:854–857
8. Gill IS, Fergany A, Klein EA (2000) Laparoscopic radical cystoprostatectomy with ileal conduit performed completely intracorporeally—the initial 2 cases. Urology 56:26–30
9. Hawasli A, Lloyd LR (1991) Laparoscopic cholecystectomy. The learning curve: report of 50 patients. Am Surg 57:542–544; discussion, 545
10. Perednia DA, Allen A (1995) Telemedicine technology and clinical applications. JAMA 273:483–484
11. Ohashi S (2002) Telesurgery, robotics and navigation surgery as an advanced technology in surgery. Rinshougeka 57:13–20
12. Rosser JC Jr, Gabriel N, Herman B, Murayama M (2001) Telementoring and teleproctoring. World J Surg 25:1438–1448
13. Link RE, Schulam PG, Kavoussi LR (2001) Telesurgery. Remote monitoring and assistance during laparoscopy. Urol Clin North Am 28:177–188
14. Buckingham RA, Buckingham RO (1995) Robots in operating theatres. BMJ 311:1479–1482

15. Drake JM, Joy M, Goldenberg A, Kreindler D (1991) Computer- and robot-assisted resection of thalamic astrocytomas in children. Neurosurgery 29:27–33
16. Mittelstadt B, Paul HA, Taylor RH, Kazanzides P, Zahars J, Williamson B (1993) Development of a surgical robot for cementless total hip replacement. Robotica 11:553–560
17. Cadiere GB, Himpens J, Germay O, Izizaw R, Degueldre M, Vandromme J, Capelluto E, Bruyns J (2001) Feasibility of robotic laparoscopic surgery: 146 cases. World J Surg 25:1467–1477
18. Rassweiler J, Frede T, Seemann O, Stock C, Sentker L (2001) Telesurgical laparoscopic radical prostatectomy. Initial experience. Eur Urol 40:75–83
19. Marescaux J, Smith MK, Fölscher D, Jamali F, Malassagne B, Leroy J (2001) Tele-robotic laparoscopic cholecystectomy: initial clinical experience with 25 patients. Ann Surg 234:1–7
20. Reichenspurner H, Damiano RJ, Mack M, Boehm DH, Gulbins H, Detter C, Meiser B, Ellgass R, Reichart B (1999) Use of the voice-controlled and computer-assisted surgical system ZEUS for endoscopic coronary artery bypass grafting. J Thorac Cardiovasc Surg 118:11–16
21. Marescaux J, Leroy J, Rubino F, Smith M, Vix M, Simone M, Mutter D (2002) Transcontinental robot-assisted remote telesurgery: feasibility and potential applications. Ann Surg 235:487–492
22. Marescaux J, Leroy J, Gagner M, Rubino F, Mutter D, Vix M, Butner SE, Smith MK (2001) Transatlantic robot-assisted telesurgery. Nature 413:379–380
23. Held G (1996) Understanding data communications, 5th edn. Sams Publishing, Indianapolis, IN, USA
24. Stallings W (1998) High-speed networks: TCP/IP and ATM design principles. Prentice-Hall, Upper Saddle River, NY, USA
25. Ushiyama T, Suzuki K, Aoki M, Takayama T, Kageyama S, Ohtawara Y, Fujita K, Uchikubo A (2003) Laparoscopic adrenalectomy using telementoring system. Nippon Hinyokika Gakkai Zasshi 94:582–586
26. Janetschek G, Bartsch G, Kavoussi LR (1998) Transcontinental interactive laparoscopic telesurgery between the United States and Europe. J Urol 160:1413
27. Sheybani EO, Sankar R (2002) ATMTN: a telemammography network architecture. IEEE Trans Biomed Eng 49:1438–1443
28. Sackier JM, Wang Y (1994) Robotically assisted laparoscopic surgery. From concept to development. Surg Endosc 8:63–66
29. Allaf ME, Jackman SV, Schulam PG, Cadeddu JA, Lee BR, Moore RG, Kavoussi LR (1998) Laparoscopic visual field. Voice vs foot pedal interfaces for control of the AESOP robot. Surg Endosc 12:1415–1418
30. Su LM, Stoianovici D, Jarrett TW, Patriciu A, Roberts WW, Cadeddu JA, Ramakumar S, Solomon SB, Kavoussi LR (2002) Robotic percutaneous access to the kidney: comparison with standard manual access. J Endourol 16:471–475
31. Satava RM (1999) Emerging technologies for surgery in the 21st century. Arch Surg 134:1197–1202
32. Kayser K, Drlicek M (1992) Visual telecommunication for expert consultation of intraoperative sections. Zentralbl Pathol 138:395–398
33. Cross SS, Burton JL, Dube AK, Feeley KM, Lumb PD, Stephenson TJ, Start RD (2002) Offline telepathology diagnosis of colorectal polyps: a study of inter-observer agreement and comparison with glass slide diagnoses. J Clin Pathol 55:452–460

34. Montironi R, Thompson D, Scarpelli M, Bartels HG, Hamilton PW, da Silva VD, Sakr WA, Weyn B, van Daele A, Bartels PH (2002) Transcontinental communication and quantitative digital histopathology via the Internet: with special reference to prostate neoplasia. J Clin Pathol 55:305–313

35. Dunn BE, Almagro UA, Choi H, Sheth NK, Arnold JS, Recla DL, Krupinski EA, Graham AR, Weinstein RS (1997) Dynamic-robotic telepathology: Department of Veteran Affairs feasibility. Hum Pathol 28:8–12

36. Kuo RL, Aslan P, Dinlenc CZ, Lee BR, Screnci D, Babayan RK, Kavoussi LR, Preminger GM (1999) Secure transmission of urologic images and records over the Internet. J Endourol 13:141–146

37. Lee SK, Peng CH, Wen CH, Huang SK, Jiang WZ (1999) Consulting with radiologists outside the hospital by using Java. Radiographics 19:1069–1075

38. Shepherd B (1999) Establishing radiologic image transmission via a transmission control protocol/Internet protocol network between two teaching hospitals in Houston. J Digit Imaging 12:88–90

39. Tachakra S, Uko Uche C, Stinson A (2002) Four years' experience of telemedicine support of a minor accident and treatment service. J Telemed Telecare 2:87–89

40. Chinnock C (1994) Virtual reality in surgery and medicine. Hosp Technol Ser 13:1–48

41. Hiatt JR, Shabot MM, Phillips EH, Haines RF, Grant TL (1996) Telesurgery. Acceptability of compressed video for remote surgical proctoring. Arch Surg 13:396–401

42. Rosser JC, Wood M, Payne JH, Fullum TM, Lisehora GB, Rosser LE, Barcia PJ, Savalgi RS (1997) Telementoring. A practical option in surgical training. Surg Endosc 11:852–855

43. Cubano M, Poulose BK, Talamini MA, Stewart R, Antosek LE, Lentz R, Nibe R, Kutka MF, Mendoza-Sagaon M (1999) Long distance telementoring: a novel tool for laparoscopy aboard the USS Abraham Lincoln. Surg Endosc 13:673–678

44. Jones JA, Johnston S, Campbell M, Miles B, Billica R (1999) Endoscopic surgery and telemedicine in microgravity: developing contingency procedures for exploratory class space flight. Urology 53:892–897

45. Satava RM (1997) Virtual reality and telepresence for military medicine. Ann Acad Med Singapore 26:118–120

46. Taniguchi E, Ohashi S (2000) Construction of a regional telementoring network for endoscopic surgery in Japan. IEEE Trans Inf Technol Biomed 4:195–199

47. Kavoussi LR, Moore RG, Partin AW, Bender JS, Zenilman ME, Satava RM (1994) Telerobotic assisted laparoscopic surgery: initial laboratory and clinical experience. Urology 44:15–19

48. Moore RG, Adams JB, Partin AW, Docimo SG, Kavoussi LR (1996) Telementoring of laparoscopic procedures: initial clinical experience. Surg Endosc 10:107–1010

49. Cheriff AD, Schulam PG, Docimo SG, Moore RG, Kavoussi LR (1996) Telesurgical consultation. J Urol 156:1391–1393

50. Schulam PG, Docimo SG, Saleh W, Breitenbach C, Moore RG, Kavoussi L (1997) Telesurgical mentoring. Initial clinical experience. Surg Endosc 11:1001–1005

51. Lee BR, Bishoff JT, Janetschek G, Bunyaratevej P, Kamolpronwijit W, Cadeddu JA, Ratchanon S, O'Kelley S, Kavoussi LR (1998) A novel method of surgical instruction: international telementoring. World J Urol 16:367–370

52. Lee BR, Caddedu JA, Janetschek G, Schulam P, Docimo SG, Moore RG, Partin AW, Kavoussi LR (1998) International surgical telementoring: our initial experience. Stud Health Technol Inform 50:41–47

53. Lee BR, Png DJ, Liew L, Fabrizio M, Li MK, Jarrett JW, Kavoussi LR (2000) Laparoscopic telesurgery between the United States and Singapore. Ann Acad Med Singapore 29:665–668

54. Micali S, Virgili G, Vannozzi E, Grassi N, Jarrett TW, Bauer JJ, Vespasiani G, Kavoussi LR (2000) Feasibility of telementoring between Baltimore (USA) and Rome (Italy): the first five cases. J Endourol 14:493–496

55. Frimberger D, Kavoussi L, Stoianovici D, Adam C, Zaak D, Corvin S, Hofstetter A, Oberneder R (2002) Telerobotic surgery between Baltimore and Munich. Urologe A 41:489–492

56. Bove P, Stoianovici D, Micali S, Patriciu A, Grassi N, Jarrett TW, Vespasiani G, Kavoussi LR (2003) Is telesurgery a new reality? Our experience with laparoscopic and percutaneous procedures. J Endourol 17:137–142

57. Rodrigues Netto N Jr, Mitre AI, Lima SV, Fugita OE, Lima ML, Stoianovici D, Patriciu A, Kavoussi LR (2003) Telementoring between Brazil and the United States: initial experience. J Endourol 17:217–220

58. Cadeddu JA, Bzostek A, Schreiner S, Barnes AC, Roberts WW, Anderson JH, Taylor RH, Kavoussi LR (1997) A robotic system for percutaneous renal access. J Urol 158:1589–1593

59. Rovetta A, Sala R (1995) Execution of robot-assisted biopsies within the clinical context. J Image Guid Surg 1:280–287

60. Koutrouvelis PG (1998) Three-dimensional stereotactic posterior ischiorectal space computerized tomography guided brachytherapy of prostate cancer: a preliminary report. J Urol 159:142–145

61. Davies BL, Hibberd RD, Ng WS, Timoney AG, Wickham JE (1991) The development of a surgeon robot for prostatectomies. Proc Inst Mech Eng [H] 205:35–38

62. Kavoussi LR, Moore RG, Adams JB, Partin AW (1995) Comparison of robotic versus human laparoscopic camera control. J Urol 154:2134–2136

63. Sheybani EO, Sankar R (2002) ATMTN: a telemammography network architecture. IEEE Trans Biomed Eng 49:1438–1443

64. Hodge JG Jr, Gostin LO, Jacobson PD (1999) Legal issues concerning electronic health information: privacy, quality, and liability. JAMA 282:1466–1471

65. Hurukawa S, Watanabe M, Ishii S, Nouga K, Kitajima M (2002) Telementor in endoscopic surgery. Rinshougeka 57:25–32

Remote Percutaneous Renal Access Using a Telesurgical Robotic System

Ben Challacombe[1], Louis Kavoussi[2], and Dan Stoianovici[2]

Summary. Urology is increasingly becoming a technology-driven specialty. With advancing technical expertise and a shift towards minimal invasion in urologic procedures, urologists are looking for ways to improve patient care using robotic and telerobotic surgical systems. Percutaneous renal access is a procedure that is ideally suited to telerobotic control, as it is a complicated task that requires precise control of the access needle through accurate initial placement and insertion without deviation. The URobotics laboratory at Johns Hopkins has developed a system for image-guided percutaneous access. An active and radiolucent needle driver, PAKY (percutaneous access to the kidney), was designed and constructed. This was then combined with the remote center of motion (RCM) robot to enable needle orientation. We describe the development of this robotic percutaneous access system from the initial laboratory trials through local clinical applications to a sequence of transatlantic telerobotic trials that have statistically proven the increased accuracy of the robot over the human hand. This has provided strong qualitative and quantitative data to support remote percutaneous renal access and telerobotic surgery in general.

Keywords. Robot, Telesurgery, Percutaneous renal access

Introduction

At a time when technology allows us to transfer information at great speeds across large distances and the public's demand for the best treatment abounds, it is hoped that in the future super-specialized surgeons will be able to operate on their patients, wherever they are in the world. Since the invention of telegraphy in 1837 and the subsequent invention of the telephone by Alexander

[1] Department of Urology, Guy's Hospital, St Thomas' Street, London, UK
[2] URobotics Laboratory, The James Buchanan Brady Urological Institute, The Johns Hopkins Medical Institutions, 600 North Wolfe Street, Suite 161, Jefferson Street Bldg, Baltimore, MD 21287-8915, USA

Graham Bell in 1875, doctors have been able to convey medical information across great distances. Telemedicine can be defined as the real-time data exchange of medical information between physicians in different locations. Telementoring describes the assistance of an experienced surgeon in a remote operation, while telesurgery implies his or her active involvement in the operation, typically through the remote control of surgical instruments. The increasing accessibility of telecommunication systems, ranging from simple telephone lines to high-bandwidth fiberoptic and satellite transmissions, has facilitated communication between physicians separated by large distances. It has been shown that surgeons are able to compensate for small transmission delays (up to about 0.5 sec) [1]. Since the development of increasingly complex surgical robots and their adaptation to be able to provide surgical assistance from remote sites, the concept of true telerobotics or telesurgery has arrived and is now reality. It has subsequently been postulated that robots may be able to perform complex surgical tasks better than their human counterparts while controlled from other locations [2].

Percutaneous Renal Surgery

In 1973, Fernstrom and Johansson [3] performed the first percutaneous operation for renal stone removal, the percutaneous pyelolithotomy. This was the first time that a percutaneous tract had been formed for the specific purpose of subsequently removing an intrarenal stone. Prior to this landmark paper, percutaneous inspection of the kidney had employed a nephrostomy tract that had been inserted at a previous open operation. In Fernstrom and Johansson's report, three patients had stones removed through a percutaneous nephrostomy under radiological control. The authors, a urologist and a radiologist, described how the percutaneous tract could be safely made and dilated using biplanar radiological guidance. The tract was progressively dilated over several days, with each catheter being exchanged for a slightly larger one until the tract was large enough for Dormia basket stone extraction.

Wickham and Kellett [4] reported the first significant series on percutaneous nephrolithotomy (PCNL) in 1981 and ensured that the technique rapidly gained worldwide approval. Despite the establishment of PCNL as one of the gold-standard procedures for removing large renal calculi, the operation itself remains technically demanding.

PCNL is a procedure that demands precise needle access to a chosen calyx as its first and most important step. Several unsuccessful attempts at needle insertion could increase the chance of patient morbidity in the form of hemorrhage, postoperative pain, and damage to adjacent structures. Hence, it is an ideal procedure to be robotically performed in an attempt to improve accuracy and decrease the risk of morbidity to the patient. There is relatively little risk of significant hemorrhage with accurate needle placement [5]. It is felt that three or fewer passes are required for safe entry into the collecting system [6], as further attempts risk significant complications. Thus, obtaining percutaneous renal access can be seen to be a complicated task requiring great skill and experience, especially in cases where the collecting system is not dilated. Some urologists have relinquished this task to interventional radiologists who use fluoroscopic, computed tomographic (CT), or ultrasound guidance, but this risks needle misplacement during the transfer back to the operating theater. Thus, there is a great need for a system to automate and facilitate this process. In addition to these benefits to the patient, telerobotic surgery, whether local or remote, can minimize or eliminate exposure of the operating surgeon to radiation.

Development of a Telesurgical Robotic System

In 1994, a group at the Imperial College in London investigated a robotic system to assist the urologist with intraoperative percutaneous renal access [7]. They employed a passive, encoded, 5 degrees of freedom (DOF) manipulator equipped with electromagnetic brakes mounted on the operating table. The access needle was manually positioned as prescribed by a computer that triangulated the calyx location from multiple C-arm images [8]. In vitro experiments evaluating system performance demonstrated a targeting accuracy of less than 1.5 mm. Nevertheless, no human trials have been performed with this system to date.

A similar system was developed at the Johns Hopkins University, which differed from the Imperial College system in that it employed an active robot (LARS) and biplanar fluoroscopy [9]. In this system, the surgeon selects the target calyx on two images, and the robot proceeds to insert the needle into the desired location. Although accuracy studies documented a margin of error of less than 1 mm, in live porcine percutaneous renal access experimentation the success rate at first attempt was only 50% [10]. Problems contributing to this included the mobility and deformability of the kidney, problems with needle deflection, and rib interference. This system, however, did prove the feasibility of performing fully automated needle placement in soft tissues. In addition, it represented another step in the evolution towards that goal in clinical practice.

The Hopkins URobotics group has developed a system for image-guided percutaneous access [11]. This system was developed on the basis that a robot should be able to reduce tremor and position the needle exactly at the required location, thus increasing safety, speed, and accuracy, while reducing radiation exposure [12]. This new system was designed to mimic the standard percutaneous renal access technique, thus providing an easy-to-use, surgeon-friendly device. The system is based on an active and radiolucent needle driver, PAKY (percutaneous access to the kidney) [13]. PAKY utilizes an axial-loaded rotational-to-translational friction transmission principle to grasp, stabilize, and advance an 18-gauge access needle into the kidney percutaneously (Fig. 1). The trocar needle used for percutaneous procedures is secured by the needle driver along its barrel near the tip in order to minimize deflection or bowing of the unsupported length

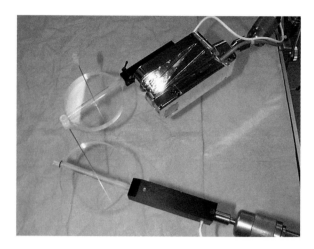

FIG. 1. PAKY stand-alone (*bottom*) and PAKY-RCM (*top*) systems

of the needle during passage through various tissue planes [14]. The needle driver is constructed with radiolucent material and thus provides an unobstructed X-ray image of the anatomical target. An electrical motor integrated into the driver's fixture makes it inexpensive to produce and permits it to be employed as a sterile disposable part [15].

Another development allowed automation of the needle orientation procedure by adding a remote center of motion (RCM) module [16]. The RCM is a compact robot adapted for surgical use [17]. It consists of a fulcrum point that is located distal to the mechanism itself, typically at the skin entry point [18]. This allows the RCM to precisely orientate a surgical instrument/needle in space while maintaining the needle tip at the skin entry point (or another specified location).

In contrast to the earlier LARS robot, the RCM employs a chain transmission rather than a parallel linkage. This permits unrestricted rotations about the RCM point and uniform rigidity of the mechanism, and eliminates singular points. The RCM can accommodate different end-effectors via an adjustment to the location of the RCM point, thus allowing the rotation to be nonorthogonal. The robot is small ($171 \times 69 \times 52$ mm box) and weighs only 1.6 kg [16], facilitating its placement within the imaging device (Fig. 2).

The needle is initially placed into the PAKY so that its tip is located at the remote center of motion. To confirm the position, the PAKY is equipped with a visible laser diode whose ray intersects the needle at the RCM point. The robot permits two motorized DOF about the RCM point (R1 and R2 on the schematic diagram) and is supported by a 7 DOF passive arm, which may be locked at the desired position by depressing a lever. A custom rigid rail allows the system to be mounted to the operating table to provide the fixed reference frame required to maintain the needle trajectory under the insertion force. Thus, the combined

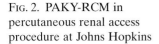

Fig. 2. PAKY-RCM in percutaneous renal access procedure at Johns Hopkins

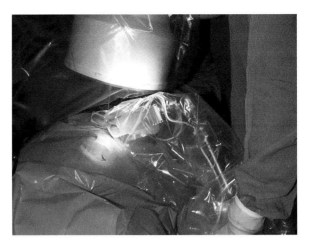

RCM-PAKY allows the needle tip to pivot about a fixed point on the skin. This allows the urologist to properly align the needle at the skin level along a selected trajectory path during fluoroscopic imaging, all by remote control, thus minimizing radiation exposure to his or her hands. The robot is therefore ideal for use in situations requiring a single entry point, such as PCNL.

An electrical impedance sensor, the "smart needle," was incorporated in the procedure needle for confirming percutaneous access through bioimpedance measurements [19]. This has been evaluated in ex vivo porcine kidneys distended with water using an 18-gauge needle, where a sharp drop in resistivity was noted from 1.9 to 1.1 ohm-m when the needle entered the collecting system [20]. The smart needle can be combined with the PAKY-RCM to detect successful entry into the renal collecting system or other percutaneous procedures via a change of resistivity.

The most recent system, AcuBot [21], augments a cartesian positioning stage and an integrated passive arm for initial positioning (Fig. 3).

These systems, in their evolving stages, have had proven feasibility, safety, accuracy, and efficacy in limited clinical trials. A more extensive trial by Su et al. validated these results [22]. In this trial, 23 patients undergoing access by the robot were compared with a contemporaneous cohort of patients undergoing access by standard techniques. The robotic system was successful in gaining access 87% of the time, with the number of attempts and time to access comparable to those with the standard technique. Furthermore, the system has been used successfully to biopsy and ablate targets in kidneys and spine and to gain percutaneous renal access in international telesurgical cases [12, 23] (see over). Although its use in humans has been limited to date, this system demonstrates great promise and has the potential to provide a mechanical platform for a completely automated percutaneous renal access.

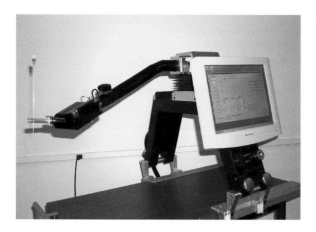

Fig. 3. The AcuBot Robot

Telesurgery

In order to perform a telesurgical operation, one must have a robot at the remote site, a data input device at the local station, and a means of transmitting the information between the sites. A telesurgery system is a combination of a video-conferencing system and a robot capable of teleportation properly customized and programmed for the surgical case.

The vital ingredient of successful telerobotic surgery lies in the speed of transfer of information from operator to robot and back again [1]. Time delay can significantly affect remote surgical performance, and if the lag time (operator-robot-operator) is more than 700 ms, the operator is unable to learn to compensate. With current high-speed connections, the delay for Earth-to-Earth connection may be of only 200 to 300 ms, which is hardly noticeable. The first telerobotic operation was performed by an Italian group, headed by Professor Rovetta [24] of Milan, who successfully performed a telerobotic prostate biopsy in 1995.

Telesurgery with the PAKY-RCM System

The PAKY-RCM arm has been successfully used as the first step in transcontinental PCNL between two countries in a few patients. On June 17, 1998, the first remote telerobotic percutaneous renal access procedure was performed between the Johns Hopkins Hospital, Baltimore, Maryland, USA, and Tor Vergata University, Rome, Italy, a distance of some 11,000 miles [23]. Remote control of the robot was accomplished over a plain old telephone system line. Video connections were established using three ISDN lines on the Italian side switched to a T1 line in the United States. The telesurgical robot was successful in terms of obtaining percutaneous access within 20 min, with two attempts to obtain entry into the collecting system.

In 2003 the group from Baltimore made a connection with a team in São Paulo, Brazil [25]. They described a laparoscopic bilateral varicocelectomy and a per-cutaneous renal access for PCNL. The technical setup consisted of a 650-MHz personal computer fitted with a Z360 video CODEC (coder/decoder) and a Z208 communication board (Zydacron, Manchester, NH, USA). This formed the core of the telesurgical station. In the PCNL patient, access to the urinary tract was achieved with the first needle pass, and percutaneous nephrolithotomy was uneventful. Blood loss was minimal, and the patient was discharged home on the second postoperative day.

Both of these initial clinical telerobotic procedures demonstrated the feasi-bility and safety of remote robotic needle access to the kidney during percuta-neous procedures. Despite these successes, there were little quantitative data to scientifically support telerobotic PCNL in terms of speed and accuracy until a series of experiments between Johns Hopkins in Baltimore and Guy's Hospital in London [26], in 2002. In the first of these, half the needle insertions (152) were performed by a robotic arm (Fig. 4) and the other half by urological surgeons. The order was decided by the toss of a coin, except for a subgroup of 30 transatlantic robotic procedures. These robotic attempts were entirely controlled by a team at Johns Hopkins via four ISDN lines for video, sound, and robot data. The technical specifications were almost identical to the previous clinical case reports, as outlined above. A successful needle insertion was confirmed by passage of either a guidewire or contrast into the collecting system of the kidney model. For the robotic procedures, the operators viewed monitors showing both the robotic arm and a fluoroscopy image of the model in real time.

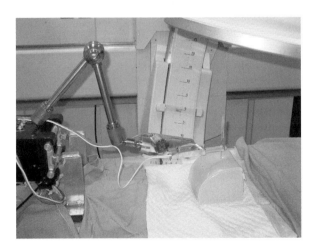

Fig. 4. PAKY-RCM during the transatlantic trial at Guy's Hospital, London

All needle attempts were successfully completed within three passes, with an interquartile range of 25 to 52 s (median, 35 s) for the human attempts compared with an interquartile range of 41 to 80 s (median, 56 s) for the robotic attempts. The robot was slower than the human operators to complete the insertions ($p < 0.001$, Mann-Whitney U test), but it was more accurate than the human operators because it made fewer attempts (the rate of success on the first attempt was 88% for the robot vs. 79% for the humans; $p = 0.046$, chi-squared test). All surgeons required fewer needle passes when using the robotic arm. The median time taken for transatlantic robotic needle insertion (59 s) was comparable to the median time taken for local robotic needle insertion (56 s), with no difference in accuracy.

In a second crossover trial [27], half of the needle insertions (30) were performed by a robotic arm in Guy's Hospital in London controlled by a team at Johns Hopkins in Baltimore via four ISDN lines; the other half of the needle insertions were controlled by the same robotic arm in the reverse direction. Again, all needle attempts were successful within two passes, with a median of 63 s for the Baltimore-to-London attempts compared with a median of 57 s for the London-to-Baltimore attempts ($p = 0.266$). There was no difference in accuracy between the trials controlled in different directions: the rate of first-pass accuracy was 84% for the Baltimore-to-London attempts, compared with 97% accuracy for the London-to-Baltimore attempts ($p = 0.103$). In comparison with the locally controlled robotic needle insertions, there was again no difference in time (median, 62 s) or accuracy (91% rate of first-pass success).

From these trials one can conclude not only that telerobotic PCNL is feasible, but also that the robot is more accurate than the human hand, since it is significantly more successful on the first attempt. In addition, the remote robotic procedures compared favorably with local robotic and human procedures. The advantage of increased accuracy is maintained in both directions, and thus remote robot-assisted PCNL may have significant advantages in terms of accuracy and hence potential patient safety.

The Future

Robotic surgery is set to become the next major revolution in modern surgery, with remote operative control becoming an increasingly significant part of this development. We have now seen the first true telerobotic surgical procedure, known as the Lindbergh operation, which involved a laparoscopic cholecystectomy between New York and Strasbourg, France [28].

It has now been confirmed that telerobotic percutaneous renal access between intercontinental sites is a feasible, reproducible, and technically achievable procedure. When a percutaneous model is used, the remote robotic needle insertion has been seen to be slightly slower than the manual insertion, but it outperforms the human operator in terms of increased accuracy. In addition, remote telerobotic access is as accurate as local telerobotic access in either transatlantic direction.

It is also anticipated that further clinical procedures involving the PAKY-RCM or similar systems can be performed from different countries, reproducing the initial results. The issues of consent and responsibility for patient care are as yet unresolved, as they are for all telerobotic procedures, but it is hoped that agreements between participating institutions will allow continued successful collaborations. With regard to cost, the computer hardware and ISDN line installation and connection are available for around $10,000, although there is an additional line usage fee of close to $1000 per hour. Despite these potential obstacles, continued interest and technological development in this field should allow increased telerobotic activity.

Remote percutaneous access and telerobotic surgery in general are particularly suited for use in large countries with remote populations. They will enable the patient of tomorrow access to the most experienced urologists wherever they are in the world, combined with the added benefit of the precision of robotic control.

Disclosure

Under licensing agreements between ImageGuide (iG) and the Johns Hopkins University (JHU), D. Stoianovici is entitled to a share of royalties received by JHU on iG's sales of products embodying the PAKY, RCM, and AcuBot technology presented in this article. Under a private license agreement, D. Stoianovici is entitled to royalties on iG's sales of products embodying the technology described in this article. D. Stoianovici and JHU own iG stock, which is subject to certain restrictions under JHU policy. D. Stoianovici is a paid consultant to iG and a paid member of the company's Scientific Advisory Board. The terms of this arrangement are being managed by the JHU in accordance with its conflict of interest policies.

Acknowledgments. The work of the URobotics lab was partially supported by grant No. 1R21CA088232-01A1 from the National Cancer Institute (NCI). The contents are solely the responsibility of the author and do not necessarily represent the official views of NCI.

References

1. Fabrizio MD, Lee BR, Chan DY, et al (2000) Effect of time delay on surgical performance during telesurgical manipulation. J Endourol 14:133–138
2. Taylor RH, Stoianovici D (2003) A survey of medical robotics in computer-integrated surgery. IEEE Trans Rob Autom 19:765–781

3. Fernstrom I, Johansson B (1976) Percutaneous pyelolithotomy. A new extraction technique. Scand J Urol Nephrol 10:257–259
4. Wickham JE, Kellett MJ (1981) Percutaneous nephrolithotomy. Br J Urol 53:297–299
5. Dunnick NR, Carson CC 3rd, Moore AV Jr, et al (1985) Percutaneous approach to nephrolithiasis. AJR Am J Roentgenol 144:451–455
6. Castaneda-Zuniga W, Coleman C, Hunter D (1986) Percutaneous nephrostomy: basic approach and fluoroscopic techniques. Thieme, New York, pp 35–44
7. Potamianos P, Davies BL, Hibberd RD (1994) Intra-operative imaging guidance for keyhole surgery: methodology and calibration, International Symposium on Medical Robotics and Computer Assisted Surgery, Pittsburgh, PA
8. Potamianos P, Davies BL, Hibberd RD (1995) Intra-operative registration for percutaneous surgery. International Symposium on Medical Robotics and Computer Assisted Surgery, Baltimore, MD
9. Bzostek A, Schreiner S, Barnes A, et al (1997) An automated system for precise percutaneous access of the renal collecting system. In: CVRMed-MRCAS. Lecture notes in computer science. Springer, pp 1205–1299
10. Caddedu JA, Bzostek A, Schreiner S, et al (1997) A robotic system for percutaneous renal access. J Urol 158:1589–1593
11. Stoianovici D (2001) URobotics—Urology Robotics at Johns Hopkins. Comput Aided Surg 6:360–369
12. Solomon SB, Patriciu A, Bohlman ME, Kavoussi LR, Stoianovici D (2002) Robotically driven interventions: a method of using CT fluoroscopy without radiation exposure to the physician. Radiology 225:277–282
13. Stoianovici D, Kavoussi LR, Whitcomb LL, et al. Friction transmission with axial loading and a radiolucent surgical needle driver. United States Patent 6,400,979, June 4
14. Stoianovici D, Cadeddu JA, Demaree RD, et al (1997) An efficient needle injection technique and radiological guidance method for percutaneous procedures. In: Lecture notes in computer science, computer vision, virtual reality and robotics in medicine— medical robotics and computer-assisted surgery (CVRMed-MRCAS'97). March 1997. Vol 1205. Springer, Grenoble, France
15. Stoianovici D, Cadeddu JA, Demaree RD, et al (1997) A novel mechanical transmission applied to percutaneous renal access. In: ASME dynamic systems and control. American Society of Mechanical Engineers, Winter Annual Meeting, Dallas, TX, November 17–18, 1997. Vol DSC Vol 61
16. Stoianovici D, Whitcomb LL, Anderson JH, Taylor RH, Kavoussi LR (1998) A modular surgical robotic system for image guided percutaneous procedures. In: Lecture notes in computer science, medical image computing and computer-assisted intervention. Vol 1496. Springer
17. Stoianovici D, Whitcomb LL, Mazilu D, Taylor RH, Kavoussi LR. Adjustable remote center of motion robotic module. United States Provisional Patent 60/354,656, Filed 02/06/02
18. Patriciu A, Stoianovici D, Whitcomb LL, et al (2000) Motion-based robotic instrument targeting under C-arm fluoroscopy. In: Lecture notes in computer science, medical image computing and computer-assisted intervention, Pittsburgh, PA, October 11–14, 2000. Vol 1935. Springer
19. Stoianovici D, Kavoussi LR, Allaf M, Jackman S. Surgical needle probe for electrical impedance measurements. United States Patent 6,337,994, January 8

20. Hernandez DJ, Sinkov VA, Roberts WW, et al (2001) Measurement of bio-impedance with a smart needle to confirm percutaneous kidney access. J Urol 166:1520–1523

21. Stoianovici D, Cleary K, Patriciu A, et al (2003) AcuBot: a robot for radiological interventions. IEEE Trans Rob Autom 19:926–930

22. Su LM, Stoianovici D, Jarrett TW, et al (2002) Robotic percutaneous access to the kidney: comparison with standard manual access. J Endourol 16:471–475

23. Bauer J, Lee BR, Stoianovici D, et al (2001) Remote percutaneous renal access using a new automated telesurgical robotic system. Telemedicine Journal and E-Health 7:341–346

24. Rovetta A, Bejczy AK, Sala R (1997) Telerobotic surgery: applications on human patients and training with virtual reality. Stud Health Technol Inform 39:508–517

25. Rodrigues Netto N Jr, Mitre AI, Lima SV, et al (2003) Telementoring between Brazil and the United States: initial experience. J Endourol 17:217–220

26. Challacombe B, Patriciu A, Glass J, et al (2003) Systematic trans-Atlantic randomised telerobotic access to the kidney: STARTRAK. Eur Urol S2

27. Challacombe B, Patriciu A, Glass J, et al (2004) Trans-Atlantic telerobotics: it cuts both ways. Eur Urol S3

28. Marescaux J, Leroy J, Gagner M, et al (2001) Transatlantic robot-assisted telesurgery. Nature 413:379–380

Radiofrequency Ablation for Percutaneous Treatment of Malignant Renal Tumors

Susumu Kanazawa[1], Toshihiro Iguchi[1], Kotaro Yasui[1],
Hidefumi Mimura[1], Tomoyasu Tsushima[2], and Hiromi Kumon[2]

Summary. We review our early experience with radiofrequency (RF) ablation of malignant renal tumors. Sixteen malignant renal tumors in 12 patients were treated. These tumors included 15 renal-cell carcinomas (RCCs) and one metastatic tumor of the retroperitoneal leiomyosarcoma. Tumor size ranged from 7 to 35 mm (mean, 24 mm). No tumor had a cystic component. Thirteen tumors were exophytic, and the other 3 tumors showed parenchymal localization. All procedures were performed with computed tomographic (CT) fluoroscopic guidance in an Interventional CT System Suite in our hospital. On the basis of the size and location of the lesion on CT scans, overlapping ablations were performed by repositioning the needle to ablate the entire tumor. In one patient whose RCC was incidentally discovered during the survey of metastatic lesions of esophageal carcinoma, transcatheter arterial chemoembolization of RCC was performed before the start of radiotherapy and chemotherapy of the esophageal carcinoma. Technical success was defined as the absence of enhancement in any area of tumor on CT or magnetic resonance (MR) images. In 15 of 16 tumors (94%), technical success was achieved. We could not achieve a complete ablation in one RCC of parenchymal localization adjacent to the renal sinus. No patient showed significant renal dysfunction after RF ablation procedures. Complications, including macro- or microhematuria, subcapsular hematoma, and pneumothorax, required only conservative observation, and all were resolved without any treatment. RF ablation for renal malignant tumor is a minimally invasive and effective treatment.

Keywords. Radiofrequency ablation, Renal-cell carcinoma, Malignant renal tumor, CT guidance, CT fluoroscopy

Percutaneous image-guided ablation with the use of radiofrequency (RF) has recently received much attention as minimally invasive therapy for solid malig-

Departments of [1]Radiology and [2]Urology, Okayama University Medical School, 2-5-1 Shikatacho, Okayama 700-8558, Japan

nancies [1–4]. Although other thermal energy sources, such as microwaves, high-intensity ultrasonography, cryotherapy, and lasers, are also used clinically, RF seems to be the most popular source, probably because of its high utility and feasibility. It has been available for treatment of primary or metastatic hepatic tumors since the early 1990s [5–7]. Recently, percutaneous RF ablation with the use of image guidance for treating tumors of the lung, bone, and kidney has been reported [8–19].

Small malignant renal tumors are being discovered with increasing frequency. They are usually discovered incidentally by abdominal ultrasound and/or computed tomography (CT). Although radical nephrectomy has been considered standard treatment for renal-cell carcinoma (RCC), partial nephrectomy is being performed increasingly as an alternative to radical nephrectomy [20, 21]. Increase in the incidence of small, incidentally found tumors has changed surgical techniques to spare normal renal parenchyma. RF ablation seems to represent a less invasive technique for treating small renal tumors while preserving renal parenchyma. In this article, we review our early experience with RF ablation of small renal malignant tumors to evaluate its efficacy.

Materials and Methods

Patients

An institutional review board approved a clinical trial of percutaneous RF ablation with CT guidance of renal malignant tumors at Okayama University Hospital in May 2002. Between May 2002 and October 2003, 12 patients, who provided informed consent, were enrolled in this study.

Sixteen malignant renal tumors in 12 patients (7 men and 5 women; mean age, 57 years; range, 23–83 years) were treated. These tumors included 15 RCCs and one metastatic tumor of the retroperitoneal leiomyosarcoma. Tumor size raged from 7 to 35mm (mean, 24mm). No tumor had a cystic component. Thirteen tumors were exophytic, and the other 3 tumors showed parenchymal localization.

The indications for RF ablation were conditions that rendered surgery highly risky because of pulmonary or cardiovascular diseases, absence of response to chemotherapy or immunotherapy, presence of a solitary kidney, or von Hippel-Lindau disease (VHL). The latter group of patients often present with RCCs at a young age and develop multiple and bilateral RCC tumors that result in multiple resections, total nephrectomy, and finally the need for dialysis [22]. Two board-certified interventional radiologists in collaboration with one experienced urologist evaluated all patients to determine their suitability for RF ablation. Thus, five patients with a solitary kidney and two patients with VHL were included in this study. In all patients, preoperative routine examination showed that the prothrombin time, partial thromboplastin time, and complete blood count were within normal limits.

RF Ablation

All ablation procedures were performed under intravenous sedation with 100µg of phentanyl citrate and local anesthesia with 1% lidocaine. Internally cooled electrodes with impedance-controlled pulse current from a 200W generator (Radionics, Burlington, MA, USA) were used for ablation (Fig. 1). All tumors were treated with a single (1- or 2-cm active tip) needle electrode. We usually started with RF energy of 20W and then gradually increased the energy by 10W every 2min. When the impedance of the tumor reached 20Ω larger than that at the beginning of ablation (the so-called breakdown) and the temperature of the tumor exceeded 60°C, we completed the ablation.

All procedures were performed with CT fluoroscopic guidance in an Interventional CT System Suite in our hospital (Figs. 2 and 3b). On the basis of the size and location of the lesion on CT scans, overlapping ablations were performed by repositioning the needle to ablate the entire tumor. In almost all cases,

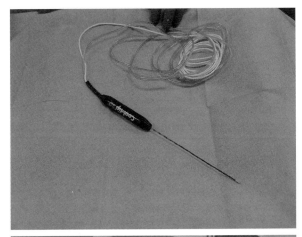

a

FIG. 1. An internally cooled electrode (**a**) with impedance-controlled pulse current from a 200-W generator (**b**) was used in ablation. We usually use an electrode with a 15-cm shaft length and a 1- or 2-cm active tip. The diameter of the electrode is 17 gauge

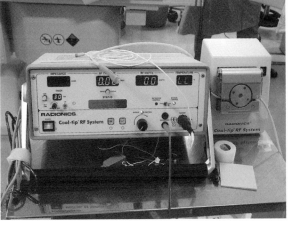

b

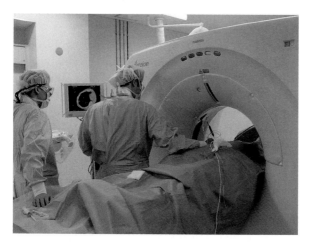

Fig. 2. Interventional computed tomographic (CT) suite provides CT fluoroscopy. An operator inserts an electrode under CT fluoroscopic guidance into the renal lesion. This suite also provides angiography equipment

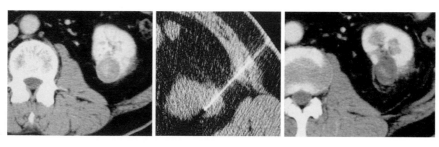

a   b,c

Fig. 3. A 60-year-old man with left renal-cell carcinoma (RCC). He had a right nephrectomy 3 years previously because of RCC. The contrast-enhanced CT scan shows an exophytic renal tumor 3 cm in diameter (a). Radiofrequency (RF) ablation with the use of an internally cooled electrode under CT fluoroscopic guidance was performed with the patient in the prone position (b). The 1-year follow-up CT scan shows complete disappearance of enhancement of the tumor (c)

the electrode was initially placed to enable ablation of the portion of the tumor neighboring on normal renal parenchyma. Ablation of this initial placement was thought to induce larger burn diameters by obstructing the cooling effect of the blood flow from the adjacent normal parenchyma. We usually repositioned a needle within 1 cm from the track of the needle positioned immediately before. If the axis of the tumor parallel to the electrode was longer than the expected burn length, overlap was obtained by pulling the electrode back for the appropriate distance and performing another ablation. At the end of the ablation procedure, dynamic CT scans of the treated kidney were performed in the Interventional CT System Suite to confirm the disappearance of enhancement of renal tumors by contrast material. If residual enhancement was observed in the tumor, further ablations were performed until the enhancement disappeared completely.

In one patient whose RCC was incidentally discovered during a survey for metastatic lesions of esophageal carcinoma, transcatheter arterial chemo-embolization of RCC was performed before the start of radiotherapy and chemotherapy of the esophageal carcinoma. After completion of 3 months of radiotherapy and chemotherapy, RF ablation of the embolized RCC was per-formed. The diameter of the tumor was 33 mm at the time of RF ablation; it had been 40 mm before embolization.

Follow-up

Follow-up CT or magnetic resonance (MR) abdominal imaging was first per-formed at 1 month and was then performed at 3, 6, and 12 months after abla-tion. The treated tumors were assessed for residual enhancement.

Technical success was defined as the absence of enhancement in any area of tumor on CT or MR images from the 1-month follow-up study. Recurrent disease was defined as new tumor enhancement after at least one imaging study had demonstrated complete eradication of enhancement.

In all patients, renal function was assessed by the value of blood urea nitro-gen (BUN), creatinine, and 24-h clearance of creatinine immediately before and after the procedure. In 12 patients, technetium-99m MAG 3 scintigraphy was also performed immediately before and after RF ablation.

Results

Technical Success

The duration of follow-up was 2 to 13 months (mean, 5.8 months). In 15 of 16 tumors (94%), technical success was achieved (Fig. 3). Among them, three lesions showed a residual enhancement at the portion adjacent to the normal renal parenchyma, and two lesions showed enhancement at the portion protruding into the renal sinus. When this was confirmed by dynamic CT scans immediately after ablation, an additional ablation was performed. After the additional abla-tion, recurrent disease was not observed in any of the patients during the follow-up period. However, we could not achieve a complete ablation in one tumor. This tumor was a RCC 35 mm in diameter located in the parenchyma adjacent to the renal sinus (Fig. 4). Although three ablations of the residual enhanced portion were performed over 12 months, absence of enhancement was not obtained.

The maximum power was 20 to 110 W (mean, 60.4 W), and the coagulation time was 2 to 50 min (mean, 11.8 min) for a total of 78 ablations.

Renal Function and Complications

No patients had significant renal dysfunction after RF ablation procedures. Technetium-99m MAG 3 scintigraphy was useful to evaluate the respective renal

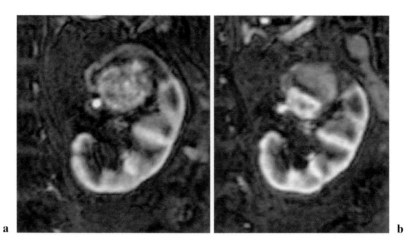

a   b

Fig. 4. A 68-year-old woman with left RCC. Left nephrectomy was avoided because of
her poor renal function. The dynamic magnetic resonance (MR) image before RF ablation shows well-enhanced tumor protruding into the renal sinus (**a**). After RF ablation,
the dynamic MR image shows disappearance of enhancement of the upper portion of the
tumor, while residual enhancement of the lower portion of the tumor is depicted (**b**)

function after RF ablation. In four patients, increase in the value of ERPF (effective renal plasma flow) of the untreated kidney immediately after the RF ablation was observed. Although this seemed to be a compensatory increase in the
renal function of the untreated kidney, no statistically significant difference was
observed.

Complications were as follows: macrohematuria in one patient, microhematuria in eight patients, perirenal or subcapsular hematoma in four patients, and
pneumothorax in one patient. These required only conservative observation, and
all were resolved without any treatment.

Discussion

Recently, the indications for RF ablation of malignancy have been rapidly
enlarged because of its feasibility and utility. Several studies have reported the
treatment of renal malignancies by RF ablation [8–11, 17–19]. According to those
papers, the complete ablation rate is as high as 79% to 100% [17–19]. Complete
ablation was reported even in an exophytic RCC 5 cm in diameter [19]. On the
other hand, in RCCs of parenchymal localization adjacent to the renal sinus,
complete ablation was sometimes difficult if the tumor diameter was smaller
than 3 cm [19]. Our results showed the same tendency. Our success rate was 94%,
although one parenchymal tumor could not be completely ablated, despite
repeated ablations. Near the renal sinus, the central portion of the kidney contains large vessels that serve as a heat sink because of the constant inflow of

blood at body temperature. However, when we ablate an exophytic tumor, the temperature conditions are different. With respect to tissue characteristics, the kidney is surrounded by fat that serves as a heat insulator. Higher ablation temperatures can be achieved and maintained in tumors that are surrounded at least in part by fat. As a result, exophytic tumors seem to be more easily treatable. Gervais et al. reported that when one is assessing a tumor for possible ablation, one can select exophytic tumors up to 5 cm in size with a high certainty that the procedure will be successful [19]. On the other hand, among tumors larger than 3 cm, those with a central component near large vessels were less likely to be treated with technical success than those without such a component. Thus, tumor location seems to be the most important factor for successful ablation of malignant renal tumors. However, even if a tumor is exophytic but located near the bowel, we must pay attention to prevent bowel perforation by burning.

We planned RF ablation with axial images from preoperative CT scans. RF ablation was then performed under CT fluoroscopic guidance. Overlapping ablations were performed by repositioning the needle to ablate the entire tumor, and we usually repositioned a needle less than 1 cm from the track of the needle positioned immediately before. By careful ablation under CT fluoroscopic guidance, we could obtain good results. However, we once performed an incomplete ablation of the caudal part of the tumor in the first ablation in one tumor. This was probably due to the underestimation of the caudal extension of the tumor by interpretation of only axial CT scan images. Sagittal, and coronal preoperative reconstruction images will reduce this kind of mistake.

We had two patients with VHL. Such patients often present with RCC at a young age and develop multiple and bilateral RCC tumors that result in multiple resections, total nephrectomy, and finally the need for dialysis [17, 18, 22]. RF ablation enables maximal maintenance of residual renal function and delays the start of dialysis. RF ablation may become the first choice for treatment of RCC in patients with VHL. Like patients with VHL, patients with a solitary kidney can obtain great benefit by RF ablation treatment when they suffer from RCC. They also need maximal maintenance of residual renal function after treatment.

Reported complications of percutaneous RF ablation include nausea, pain, hematuria, and hematoma [17, 19]. Although a case of ureteral stenosis causing renal dysfunction after RF ablation was reported [19], no other severe complications have been reported in the previous studies. There were no severe complications among the patients in our study. Among five patients in our series with a solitary kidney, no renal dysfunction was observed after RF ablation. RF ablation is a safe and feasible treatment for RCC.

Percutaneous RF ablation should be compared with partial nephrectomy, i.e., nephron-sparing surgery. Uzoo et al. [20] described the complication rates and outcomes of nephron-sparing surgical procedures in a review of reports of these procedures. The survival data for nephron-sparing surgical procedures are similar to those for radical nephrectomy. The rate of major complications ranged from 4% to 30% in nine series, with a cumulative total of 155 (13.7%) complications in 1129 procedures. The reported results of RF ablation, including our study, are favorable compared with the results of partial nephrectomy.

In conclusion, RF ablation for RCC is a minimally invasive and effective treatment. It will be able to replace partial nephrectomy for the treatment of RCC in patients who are at high risk during anesthesia and surgery, those with a solitary kidney, and those with VHL.

References

1. Dodd GD III, Soulen MC, Kane RA, Livraghi T, Lees WR, Yamashita Y, Gillams AR, Karahan OI, Rhim H (2000) Minimally invasive treatment of malignant hepatic tumors: at the threshold of a major breakthrough. Radiographics 20:9–27
2. Gazelle GS, Goldberg SN, Solbiati L, Livraghi T (2000) Tumor ablation with radio-frequency energy. Radiology 217:633–646
3. McGahan JP, Dodd GD (2001) Radiofrequency ablation of the liver: current status. AJR 176:3–16
4. Goldberg SN, Gazelle GS, Mueller PR (2000) Thermal ablation therapy for focal malignancy: a unified approach to underlying principles, techniques, and diagnostic imaging guidance. AJR 174:323–331
5. Rossi S, DiStasi M, Bucarini E, Quaretti P, Garbagnati F, Squassante L, Paties CT, Silverman DE, Buscarini L (1996) Percutaneous RF interstitial thermal ablation in the treatment of hepatic cancer. AJR 167:759–768
6. Livraghi T, Goldberg SN, Lazzarini S, Meloni F, Solbiati L, Gazelle GS (1999) Small hepatocellular carcinoma: treatment with radio-frequency ablation versus ethanol injection. Radiology 210:655–661
7. Curley SA, Izzo F, Derlia P, Ellis LM, Granchi J, Vallone P, Fiore F, Pignata S, Daniele B, Cremona F (1999) Radiofrequency ablation of unresectable primary and metastatic hepatic malignancies: results in 123 patients. Ann Surg 161:599–600
8. Zlotta AR, Wildshutz T, Raviv G, Peny MO, van Gansbeke D, Noel JC, Schulman CC (1997) Radiofrequency interstitial tumor ablation (RITA) is a possible new modality for treatment of renal cancer: ex vivo and in vivo experience. J Endourol 11:251
9. McGovern FJ, Wood BJ, Goldberg SN, Mueller PR (1999) Radiofrequency ablation of renal cell carcinoma via image guided needle electrodes. J Urol 161:599–600
10. Gervais DA, McGovern FJ, Wood BJ, Goldberg SN, McDougal WS, Mueller PR (2000) Radiofrequency ablation of renal cell carcinoma: early clinical experience. Radiology 217:665–672
11. Walther MC, Shawker TH, Libutti SK, Lubensky I, Choyke PL, Venzon D, Linehan WM (2000) A phase 2 study of radio frequency interstitial tissue ablation of localized renal tumors. J Urol 163:1424–1427
12. Dupuy DE, Zagoria RJ, Akerly W, Mayo-Smith WW, Kavanagh PV, Safran H (2000) Percutaneous RF ablation of malignancies in the lung. AJR 174:57–60
13. Zagoria RJ, Chen MY, Kavanaugh PV, Torti FM (2001) Radio frequency ablation of lung metastasis from renal cell carcinoma. J Urol 165:1827–1828
14. Abraham J, Fojo T, Wood BJ (2000) Radiofrequency ablation of metastatic lesions in adrenocortical cancer. Ann Intern Med 133:312–313
15. Wood BJ, Bates S (2001) Radiofrequency thermal ablation of a splenic metastasis. J Vasc Interv Radiol 12:261–263

16. Callstrom MR, Charboneau JW, Goetz MP, Rubin J, Wong GY, Sloan JA, Novotny PJ, Lewis BD, Welch TJ, Farrell MA, Maus TP, Lee RA, Reading CC, Petersen IA, Pickett DD (2002) Painful metastases involving bone: feasibility of percutaneous CT- and US-guided radiofrequency ablation. Radiology 224:87–97
17. Pavlovich CP, McClellan MW, Choyke PL, Pautler SE, Chang R, Linehan WM, Wood BJ (2002) Percutaneous radio frequency ablation of small renal tumors: initial results. J Urol 167:10–15
18. de Baere T, Kuoch V, Smayra T, Dromain C, Cabrera T, Court B, Roche A (2002) Radio frequency ablation of renal cell carcinoma: preliminary clinical experience. J Urol 167:1961–1964
19. Gervais DA, McGovern FJ, Arellano RS, McDougal WS, Mueller PR (2003) Renal cell carcinoma: clinical experience and technical success with radio-frequency ablation of 42 tumors. Radiology 226:417–424
20. Uzzo RC, Novick AC (2001) Nephron sparing surgery for renal tumors: indications, techniques and outcomes. J Urol 166:6–18
21. Herring JC, Enquist EG, Chernoff A, Linehan WM, Choyke PL, Walther MM (2001) Parenchymal sparing surgery in patients with hereditary renal cell carcinoma: 10-years experiences. J Urol 165:771–781
22. Choyke PL, Glenn GM, Walther MM, Zbar B, Weiss GH, Alexander RB, Hayes WS, Long JP, Thakore KN, Linehan WM (1992) The natural history of renal lesions in von Hippel-Lindau disease: a serial CT study in 28 patients. AJR 159:1229–1234

High-Intensity Focused Ultrasound for Noninvasive Renal Tumor Thermoablation

A. Häcker[1], M.S. Michel[1], and K.U. Köhrmann[2]

Summary. The conviction that the presence of a renal-cell carcinoma does not require the entire organ to be removed allows new therapeutic methods to be envisaged that involve only local tissue ablation, rather than the complete removal of the organ. The trend toward minimally invasive options in the management of renal tumors has prompted interest in energy-based ablation techniques as a possible alternative to radical or partial nephrectomy in selected patients. Cryoablation, radiofrequency interstitial tumor ablation, microwave thermotherapy, and high-intensity focused ultrasound (HIFU) are among such techniques. HIFU has emerged as the least invasive of the possible tumor-ablation methods. The present review addresses the current literature on experimental and clinical application of HIFU for extracorporeal thermoablation of renal tumors.

Keywords. Renal-cell carcinoma, Minimally invasive therapy, High-intensity focused ultrasound

Introduction

Due to the widespread use of ultrasound, abdominal computed tomography (CT), and magnetic resonance imaging (MRI), renal tumors are being detected incidentally at increasing rates [1]. Typically, these tumors tend to be small, with lower stages yielding better survival outcomes than tumors diagnosed in symptomatic patients [2]. Surgical techniques for the treatment of locally confined renal tumors have changed drastically. Nephron-sparing surgery has gained

[1]Department of Urology, University Hospital Mannheim, Faculty of Clinical Medicine Mannheim, Ruprecht-Karls-University Heidelberg, Theodor-Kutzer-Ufer 1-3, 68135 Mannheim, Germany
[2]Theresienkrankenhaus Mannheim, Barsermannstraße 1, 68165 Mannheim, Faculty of Clinical Medicine Mannheim, Ruprecht-Karls-University, Mannheim, Germany

acceptance as an alternative to radical nephrectomy for treatment of renal tumors less than 4 cm in diameter [3, 4]. At the same time, the use of laparoscopy has resulted in decreased morbidity for patients undergoing renal extirpative surgery. Laparoscopic partial nephrectomy is a viable option in appropriately selected patients [5]. However, hemostasis following tumor excision remains an ongoing challenge. In an effort to optimize hemostasis in nephron-sparing minimally invasive surgery, as well as to further decrease the invasiveness of renal surgery through the use of percutaneous techniques, energy-based abla-tion techniques such as cryoablation, radiofrequency ablation (RFA), interstitial laser ablation, microwave thermotherapy, and high-intensity focused ultrasound (HIFU) have been introduced. Furthermore, patients who are poor surgical can-didates and those with hereditarily based renal tumors who are at risk for mul-tiple renal operations would benefit from a less invasive treatment modality that avoids surgical morbidity and potentially better preserves renal function.

HIFU has the potential to be the least invasive of the currently available tumor-ablation methods, since an energy source does not need to be introduced directly into the tumor. The present chapter addresses the current literature on experimental and clinical application of HIFU for noninvasive treatment of renal tumors.

What Is HIFU?

High-intensity focused ultrasound (HIFU) is also known as pyrotherapy, ultrasound ablation, and focused ultrasound surgery. The aim of this technique is "contactless" destruction of defined parts of an organ by extracorporeally applied ultrasound energy. If the ultrasound beam carries sufficient energy and is brought into a tight focus within the body, the energy within the focal volume can cause a local rise in temperature, resulting in a sharply demarcated thermal tissue necrosis (a "lesion"). Surrounding or overlying tissues are not damaged. The ability to cause cell death in a volume of tissue distant from the ultrasound source makes HIFU an attractive option for development as a noninvasive surgical tool.

History of HIFU

In 1942, the first work to consider potential applications of HIFU was published by Lynn and colleagues [6]. William Fry was the first researcher to produce lesions in the living tissue of cat brains [7, 8]. Frank Fry subsequently treated patients with Parkinson's disease and other neurological conditions [9]. Research into the use of HIFU in neurosurgery continued during the 1950s and 1960s [10–13], but practical and technological limitations restricted their progress. In recent years, there have been many investigations of the potential applications of HIFU across the spectrum of clinical application, e.g., the eye

[14], prostate (benign prostate hyperplasia and cancer [15, 16]), liver [17], and bladder [18].

More recently, HIFU trials on the kidney were performed. The tests carried out by Vallancien in 1992 [19, 20] revealed that, in principle, ablation of kidney tissue by means of focused ultrasound is possible. Thus far, clinical application of HIFU for the treatment of renal tumors has only been experimental in nature. To date, only a few patients have been included in feasibility studies of the treatment of renal-cell carcinoma [21, 22].

Technical Principles

Generally, the components of an HIFU system include a transducer to generate and focus ultrasound waves; an imaging device, usually a standard imaging ultrasound probe that can be placed in-line with the HIFU transducer to monitor the treatment under real-time conditions; a coupling device, such as a water bath or water cushion, to provide an interface for transmission of ultrasound energy from transducer to patient; a housing or gantry for the HIFU device; and a central computing unit from which the operator can control the treatment parameters. These control parameters are the power output, number of pulses, pulse duration, duration between pulses, focal length, and treatment volume.

Ultrasound waves are generated by high-frequency (0.5 to 10 MHz) vibration of a piezoelectric or piezoceramic transducer. They are focused by a spherically arranged acoustic lens or parabolic reflectors into a small, discrete region, the focal point. Ultrasound is coupled by degassed water between the source and patient's skin. Because of the comparable acoustic properties of water and tissue, the sound waves should penetrate the skin and further precursor tissue with only slight absorption and reflection. The power density of the converging ultrasound increases as it approaches the focal point.

The action of focused ultrasound on tissue results in thermal and nonthermal effects (cavitations, acoustic streaming, and oscillatory motion). Evidence also exists that HIFU injures blood vessels less than 2 cm from the focal zone, inducing a secondary ischemic necrosis of target tissue [23–29].

Tissue is rapidly heated to temperatures between 65° and 100°C, causing irreversible cell damage and thermal coagulative necrosis (thermal effect). There is a steep temperature gradient between the focus and neighboring tissue, which is demonstrated by the sharp demarcation between the volume of necrotic cells (lesion) and normal surrounding cells on histologic examination [30]. Acoustic cavitation is complex and unpredictable, but the end result is also cell necrosis induced through a combination of mechanical stresses and thermal injury. Cavitation is caused by a process in which bubbles develop and acutely increase in size to the point at which resonance is achieved. When the bubbles suddenly collapse, high pressures, ranging from 20,000 to 30,000 bars, develop and damage nearby cells.

The focal region is a cigar-shaped three-dimensional zone with its long axis perpendicular to the axis of wave propagation. The dimensions of the focal zone depend on the frequency and the geometry of the source; they are on the order of 10 to 50 mm in length and 1 to 5 mm in diameter. A larger volume of tissue can be ablated by sequentially shifting the focal zone by incremental movements of the transducer combined with adjustment of the focal length. The extent of tissue ablation is approximately that of the physical focal zone, but it can be controlled within a limited range by the power and duration of the ultrasound pulses [31]. By scanning the target using multiple pulses, larger areas of tissue can be ablated.

In clinical application, an important factor is the ability to monitor treatment accurately. This is achieved by using real-time ultrasound [15, 16, 32] or MRI [33]. HIFU treatment of kidney tissue can be monitored under real-time conditions by standard imaging ultrasound probes placed in line with the therapeutic HIFU transducer. The position of the therapeutic focus can therefore be identified on the diagnostic image. The extent of the treatment can be monitored by recording posttreatment gray-scale changes on the diagnostic images. However, the use of ultrasound for imaging lesions to determine precise targeting of tissue destruction is limited. Several groups [34–36] have similarly described the limitations of ultrasound in demonstrating detectable tissue changes during or following the creation of lesions. Ultrasound is also obstructed by bone and air-filled viscera. Because it is important to identify the position of such structures relative to the therapeutic beam, this is an advantage of ultrasound for real-time monitoring. Additional imaging modalities, such as duplex Doppler, CT, and MRI, applied in an online thermometry system, are therefore necessary to target the tumor precisely and to monitor the ablation effect on-line. These new techniques are still under development and investigation. MRI has the advantage of better image quality and the ability to monitor temperature. However, it is expensive and has lower spatial resolution. Today, no device exists for the treatment of renal tumors under MRI guidance.

Because of movement of the kidney during breathing, tumor localization and targeting can be difficult [34]. Watkin et al. [35] reported a poor ability to target renal lesions while using HIFU; only 67% of total shots fired were detected in the target area. When general anesthesia is used, ventilation can be stopped briefly, thus preventing movement of the kidney during application of ultrasound. General anesthesia is also required for managing pain when high energy levels are applied. However, HIFU treatments without general anesthesia have been described in the literature [22, 37].

Morphology of Lesions in the Kidney

Acoustic energy absorbed by tissue and thereby converted to heat induces coagulation necrosis within the focus. The morphological characteristics of the lesion change with the applied energy and the time of follow-up.

Immediately after ultrasound exposure with low energy levels, the lesion sometimes cannot be detected macroscopically. Even microscopy only shows an area that is less strongly stained by periodic acid-Schiff, without changes in the cellular structure [38, 39]. Ultrastructural examination of the kidney has revealed damage to organelles within the first couple of hours. The initial healing process indicated the presence of these discrete lesions. Medium energy levels induced a sharp lesion that was macroscopically detectable 1 h after HIFU treatment and that was demarcated within the next few days [40]. Focusing on the renal corticomedullary border resulted in pronounced streaky bleeding of the medulla. Macroscopic and microscopic lesions appeared to be less extensive in the cortex. Nevertheless, focusing directly on the cortex also induced a distinct defect in this area. Histologically, acute changes involved epithelial displacement and epithelial destruction of the affected tubuli. Subsequently, the stroma collapsed, revealing empty medullar tubuli and ducts with slight fibroblastic activity at the margins [40].

Köhrmann et al. [41] applied HIFU to healthy kidney tissue of 24 patients immediately before nephrectomy. In 19 of the 24 cases, hemorrhage or necrosis was detected macroscopically. Histologically, interstitial hemorrhages and fiber rupture, as well as collagen fiber shrinkage with eosinophilia, were detected in the focal area. Chapelon et al. [42] studied the effects of HIFU on rat and canine kidneys (no tumor treatment) and demonstrated lesions consistent with coagulative necrosis or cavitation, depending on the duration and intensity of ultrasound. The lesion size also varied, depending on the acoustic intensity and the number of firings. Adams et al. [34] noted that, histologically, affected cells demonstrated pale eosinophilic cytoplasm and separation from one another. At the periphery of the lesions, areas of hemorrhage were noted in close proximity to normal-appearing tissue. Susani et al. [39] treated healthy and tumorous tissue in two patients with renal tumors before performing radical nephrectomy. Two renal-cell tumors were excluded from the study because the great amount of tumor necrosis did not allow the target zone to be identified. Clearly demarcated necrosis became hemorrhagic and was later replaced by granulation tissue. The size and location of the lesions corresponded exactly to the previously determined target areas.

Research Studies

In 1992, Chapelon et al. [42] studied the effects of HIFU on rat and canine kidneys (no tumor treatment) and demonstrated precise lesions consistent with coagulative necrosis or cavitation, depending on the duration and intensity of ultrasound and the number of firings. Lesions of varying sizes were reported in 10 out of 16 treated animals (63%). However, in 13 out of 16 dogs (81%), lesions occurred in the abdominal organs (spleen, colon, lung, and pancreas). This finding was believed to be due to misfocusing on the target organ. Some improvement was achieved with the use of an ultrasound bidimensional scanner.

In 1996, Adams and colleagues [34] treated implanted VX-2 tumors in rabbit kidneys with the Sonablate transrectal system through surgical exposure as well as transcutaneously. In phase 1 of this experimental study, focused ultrasound was applied after exposing the kidney by direct contact of the source to the kidney. At 4 h, seven of nine insonated tumors showed macroscopic evidence of ablation. According to histologic examination, in all nine rabbits a well-defined area of renal and tumor tissue was damaged, corresponding to the chosen regions. Tissue destruction was characterized by eosinophilic cytoplasm and separated cells surrounded by hemorrhage. The area immediately adjacent to the targeted tissue was apparently normal. In phase 2, ultrasound was applied through the shaved flank skin. Thus, insufficient clarity of tumor imaging was explained by indirect extracorporeal application. A week later, four rabbits showed skin burns, but there were no injuries to adjacent organs. Only seven of the nine kidneys showed gross or histological tissue ablation. After this longer follow-up, nuclei were absent and the cytoplasm was pale pink in the damaged cells. Lymphocytes had infiltrated from the border of the damaged area. Furthermore, coagulative necrosis, including mineralization and tubular atrophy, was noted. Limited tumor localization on 4 MHz diagnostic ultrasound and kidney movement due to ventilation were considered reasons for insufficient ablation by percutaneous ultrasound. By the use of power Doppler ultrasound after HIFU to a $10 \times 10 \times 18$ mm area, a zone of tumor destruction was histologically demonstrated in all animals without severe side effects on renal function [43].

Watkin and associates [35] reported a poor ability to target renal tissue in pigs with the use of HIFU transcutaneously; only 67% of total shots fired were detected in the target area. Finally, Daum et al. [44] accurately created seven 0.5×0.5 cm^2 lesions in the kidneys of two pigs in vivo.

In a large-animal model, Paterson et al. [45] tested an HIFU probe for laparoscopic renal partial ablation and demonstrated its feasibility and safety. Pathological examination at 14 days revealed reproducible, homogeneous, and complete tissue necrosis throughout the whole volume of the lesion, with sharp demarcation from adjacent normal tissue.

Clinical Application

When treating healthy kidneys of eight patients with extracorporeally applied HIFU in a phase 1 study, Vallancien et al. [19] did not observe any significant changes in the usual laboratory parameters, except for a transient increase in creatine phosphokinase after a long pulse. Side effects included skin burns. Köhrmann et al. [41] applied HIFU to healthy kidney tissue of 24 patients ₂immediately before nephrectomy. In 19 out of the 24 cases, hemorrhage or necrosis was detected macroscopically. Histologically, interstitial hemorrhages and fiber rupture, as well as collagen fiber shrinkage with eosinophilia, were detected in the focal area.

In a phase 2 study, Vallancien et al. [19] treated four patients with T2-T3 renal tumors with HIFU 2, 6, 8, and 15 days before they underwent nephrectomy. Histological examination of the treated kidneys revealed a coagulation necrosis in the targeted tumor area. In two cases, a small edema formed in the perirenal fat tissue during surgery. No subcapsular or perirenal hematomas were noted. The muscle wall (lumbar incision) was normal in all cases, and there were no lesions of the adjacent organs (colon, inferior vena cava, duodenum, ureter, and renal pelvis). During operations performed on days 2 or 3, a clearly demarcated necrotic area was detected, corresponding to the selected volume. No adverse systemic effects were observed. Two patients had localized first-degree and third-degree skin burns.

Köhrmann and colleagues [21] recently reported on a patient with three renal tumors who underwent HIFU in three sessions under general or sedation anesthesia and who was followed by clinical examinations and MRI for 6 months. After HIFU treatment, MRI indicated necrosis in the two tumors of the lower pole of the kidney within 17 and 48 days. The necrotic area in these two tumors shrunk thereafter within 6 months (tumor 1 shrank from 2.3 cm, as shown in Fig. 1, to 0.8 cm, as shown in Fig. 2; tumor 2 shrank from 1.4 cm, as shown in Fig. 1, to 1.1 cm, as shown in Fig. 3). Unfortunately, one tumor in the upper pole (2.8 cm) was inadequately treated because of absorption of ultrasound energy by the interposed ribs. During one session, a skin burn of grade 2 occurred.

Wu et al. [22] reported on their preliminary experience using HIFU for the treatment of patients with advanced-stage renal malignancy. HIFU treatment (median hours of therapy, 5.4; range, 1.5 to 9) was performed in 12 patients with advanced-stage renal-cell carcinoma and 1 patient with colon cancer metastasized to the kidney (median tumor size, 8.7 cm; range, 2 to 15). All patients under-

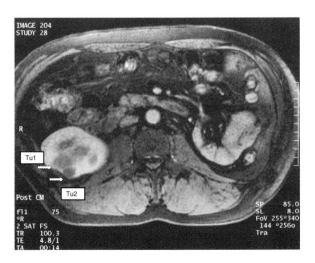

FIG. 1. Before HIFU application: two tumors in the lower pole of the kidney

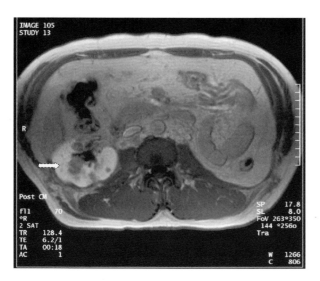

Fig. 2. Six months after HIFU treatment: shrinking of tumor 1

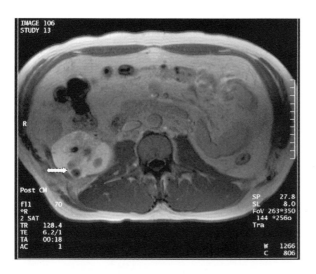

Fig. 3. Six months after HIFU treatment: shrinking of tumor 2

went HIFU treatment safely, including 10 who had partial tumor ablation and 3 who had complete ablation. After HIFU, hematuria disappeared in 7 of 8 patients and flank pain of presumed malignant origin disappeared in 9 of 10 patients. The postoperative images showed decrease in or absence of tumor blood supply in the treated region and significant shrinkage of the ablated tumor. Of the 13 patients, 7 died (median survival, 14.1 months; range, 2 to 27) and 6 were still alive after a median follow-up of 18.5 months (range, 10 to 27). A minor skin burn was observed in the first patient, which had healed 2 weeks after HIFU.

Complications, Safety, and Oncological Efficacy

HIFU is a relatively safe technique. Potential risks include urine extravasation, urinary obstruction, hemorrhage, thrombosis and hematomas, abscess, and dysfunction of the kidney and the tissue through which the waves pass. Up to now, none of these has been reported in association with the procedure.

As described above, skin burns are common side effects [21]. They occur because of absorption of ultrasound energy at the interface between two materials that have different attenuation properties. Soft tissues and water have similar attenuation values, so ultrasound waves propagate well, with minimal absorption, through these. The greatest clinically relevant attenuation occurs at the level of the skin; thus, enough energy can be absorbed by skin over the treatment site to result in second and third degree burns. Taking Köhrmann's studies together, three cases of skin burns of grade 3 were observed in 29 treated patients [46].

Because ultrasound energy is not completely transferred to thermal and mechanical energy (cavitation effects), there is a possibility that cells will mobilize, causing cancer cells to enter the circulation and promote metastasis. In various studies, no evidence of metastases has been reported. Chapelon and associates [47] determined the impact of HIFU on the development of metastases of experimental prostate cancer. In the control population, 28% of the animals developed distant metastases, whereas in the HIFU-treated animals, this percentage dropped to 16%. Similar findings were reported by Oosterhof and colleagues [48] using a T-6 Dunning R3327 rat prostate cancer subline. Metastases were seen in 23% of the HIFU-treated animals, as compared with 25% of the sham-treated animals (difference not statistically significant). From these data, it can be concluded that HIFU applied to cancer tissue does not accelerate the development of distant metastases.

HIFU is a noninvasive technique. It does not allow accurate pathological tissue diagnosis, staging, and grading of the renal mass, which determine the prognosis of the patient. Therefore, biopsy of perirenal fat and of the renal mass is promoted by some investigators [49, 50] for precise pathological diagnosis of the renal lesions (benign or malignant), which is critical for determining appropriate clinical and radiological follow-up. However, renal biopsy prior to treatment can be fraught with inaccuracies. In a prospective analysis of 100 renal lesions, Dechet et al. [51] reported nondiagnostic rates for CT and needle biopsy of 20% and 31%, respectively, and a specificity for both of 20%. According to this study, accurate preoperative pathological diagnosis using needle biopsy is critical.

Radiographic follow-up is necessary for tumor control. Immediate postoperative and long-term efficacy is assessed by the radiographic appearance of lesions at various intervals. For renal cryoablation [52], radiographic response criteria can be defined as initial evidence of infarction and hemorrhage, subsequent obliteration or reduction in size of the renal mass, and absence of growth on radiological follow-up examinations. Atypical enhancement on CT or MRI should not be considered a failure unless it is associated with persistence or growth of the mass.

In order to document the HIFU-induced thermolesions in renal tumors, Köhrmann et al. [21] performed MRI using gadolinium as the contrast medium [53]. The initial effects of HIFU were identified by MRI 2 days after treatment of the first tumor as a minimal increase in signal, similar to that caused by a hemorrhage, becoming demarcated as colliquative necrosis in the next 2 weeks. In the second tumor, delayed demarcation of necrosis occurred only after 48 days. In the third treated tumor, no lesion was seen (see above). In the study performed by Vallancien et al. [20], CT in two patients who underwent nephrectomy after thermotherapy revealed a zone with reduced density, corresponding to the treated area.

Indications

The use of HIFU for renal tumors is considered investigational. Follow-up data are rare. It is primarily useful for treating such lesions in patients with comorbidities that preclude a major surgical procedure, such as partial open or laparoscopic nephrectomy. Limited data exist on the precise anatomical characteristics that are amenable to ablative techniques (lesion size, location within the kidney, and proximity to the collecting system and the renal hilum). At present, no substantial clinical experience with HIFU for renal tumor ablation exists. It is still unclear what size or location of tumor will be amenable to this form of therapy. From our experience, the majority of candidates are those with small (less than 2 cm), dorsal and lateral exophytic lesions that are located away from the collecting system and distant from the bowel. Application of HIFU to the gas-filled bowel has a high risk of perforation necrosis of this organ. General contraindications are coagulopathy or a completely intrarenal, centrally located tumor near the renal sinus or hilum, as injury to the collecting system may result.

To date, there is no proof that HIFU destroys kidney tumors completely and permanently. Therefore, HIFU treatment of kidney tumors still has to be classified as experimental.

Conclusions

HIFU for treatment of renal tumors is being introduced as a new nephron-sparing approach in an attempt to minimize operation time, morbidity, and time to full recovery. The majority of candidates are those with small, peripheral lesions that are located away from the collecting system and the bowel. Nevertheless, inclusion criteria based on the size, location, and type of treatable lesions and patient selection are evolving.

Reliable, reproducible, and complete eradication of tumor tissue with surrounding normal renal parenchyma needs to be ensured. If HIFU, as a noninvasive ablative technique, is to gain acceptance as a nephron-sparing approach, it should have demonstrable equivalent efficacy and reduced morbidity as compared with open partial and radical nephrectomy. The limitations of HIFU in experimental and clinical studies include incomplete ablation, requiring multiple treatments to ablate the renal lesion completely. Until now, no large series with long-term results confirming the curative efficacy of HIFU for the treatment of renal tumors has been conducted. Existing studies are limited to animals, small series of patients with short-term follow-up, or case reports.

HIFU is a promising but presently experimental procedure. It will achieve routine clinical application when technical problems concerning visualization of the target organ and lesion, precise control of lesion size, complete ablation of the tumor mass, and reduction in side effects (skin burns) have been resolved. The objectives of further developments are to optimize ultrasound coupling and to provide on-line ablation evidence to ensure complete tumor ablation. At this time, HIFU should be reserved for selected patients in well-designed clinical studies.

References

1. Pantuck A, Zisman A, Belldegrun A (2001) The changing natural history of renal cell carcinoma. J Urol 166:1611–1623
2. Luciani LG, Cestari R, Tallarigo C (2000) Incidental renal cell carcinoma—age and stage characterisation and clinical implications: study of 1092 patients (1982–1997). Urology 56:58–62
3. Uzzo RG, Novick AC (2001) Nephron sparing surgery for renal tumors: indications, techniques and outcomes. J Urol 166:6–18
4. Fergany AF, Hafez KS, Novick AC (2000) Long-term results of nephron sparing surgery for localized renal cell carcinoma: 10-year followup. J Urol 163:442–445
5. Janetschek G, Daffner P, Peschel R, Bartsch G (1998) Laparoscopic nephron sparing surgery for small renal cell carcinoma. J Urol 159:1152–1155
6. Lynn J, Zwemer R, Chick A, Miller DL (1942) A new method for the generation and use of focused ultrasound in experimental biology. J Gen Physiol 26:179–193
7. Fry WJ, Mosberg WH, Barnard JW, Fry FJ (1954) Production of focal destructive lesions in the central nervous system with ultrasound. J Neurosurg 11:471–478
8. Fry W, Barnard J, Fry F, Krumins R, Brennan J (1955) Ultrasonic lesions in the mammalian central nervous system. Science 122:517–518
9. Fry FJ, Ades HW, Fry WJ, Mosberg WH Jr, Barnard JW (1958) Precision high-intensity focusing ultrasonic machines for surgery. Am J Phys Med 37:152–156
10. Ballantine HT Jr, Bell E, Manlapaz J (1960) Progress and problems in the neurological applications of focused ultrasound. J Neurosurg 17:858–876
11. Warwick R, Pond J (1968) Trackless lesions in nervous tissues produced by high-intensity focused ultrasound (high-frequency mechanical waves). J Anat 102:387–405
12. Lele PP (1966) Concurrent detection of the production of ultrasonic lesions. Med Biol Eng 4:451–456
13. Lele PP (1967) Production of deep focal lesions by focused ultrasound—current status. Ultrasonics 5:105–112

14. Haut J, Colliac JP, Falque L, Renard Y (1990) Indications and results of Sonocare (ultrasound) in the treatment of ocular hypertension. A preliminary study of 395 cases (in French). Ophtalmologie 4:138–141
15. Madersbacher S, Schatzl G, Djavan B, Stulnig T, Marberger M (2000) Long-term outcome of transrectal high-intensity focused ultrasound therapy for benign prostatic hyperplasia. Eur Urol 37:687–694
16. Chaussy C, Thuroff S (2003) The status of high-intensity focused ultrasound in the treatment of localized prostate cancer and the impact of a combined resection. Curr Urol Rep 4:248–252
17. Gignoux BM, Scoazec JY, Curiel L, Beziat C, Chapelon JY (2003) High-intensity focused ultrasonic destruction of hepatic parenchyma (in French). Ann Chir 128:18–25
18. Watkin NA, Morris SB, Rivens IH, Woodhouse CR, ter Haar GR (1996) A feasibility study for the non-invasive treatment of superficial bladder tumours with focused ultrasound. Br J Urol 78:715–721
19. Vallancien G, Harouni M, Veilon B, Mombet A, Prapotnich D, Brisset JM, Bougaran J (1992) Focused extracorporeal pyrotherapy: feasibility study in man. J Endourol 6:173–181
20. Vallancien G, Chartier-Kastler E, Bataille N, Chopin D, Harouni M, Bourgaran J (1993) Focused extracorporeal pyrotherapy. Eur Urol 23(Suppl 1):48–52
21. Köhrmann KU, Michel MS, Gaa J, Marlinghaus E, Alken P (2002) High-intensity focused ultrasound as noninvasive therapy for multilocal renal cell carcinoma: case study and review of the literature. J Urol 167:2397–2403
22. Wu F, Wang ZB, Chen WZ, Bai J, Zhu H, Qiao TY (2003) Preliminary experience using high-intensity focused ultrasound for the treatment of patients with advanced stage renal malignancy. J Urol 170:2237–2240
23. Chen L, ter Haar G, Hill CR, Dworkin M, Carnochan P, Young H, Bensted JP (1993) Effect of blood perfusion on the ablation of liver parenchyma with high-intensity focused ultrasound. Phys Med Biol 38:1661–1673
24. Hynynen K, Chung AH, Colucci V, Jolesz FA (1996) Potential adverse effects of high-intensity focused ultrasound exposure on blood vessels in vivo. Ultrasound Med Biol 22:193–201
25. Vaezy S, Martin R, Yaziji H, Kaczkowski P, Keilman G, Carter S, Caps M, Chi EY, Bailey M, Crum L (1998) Hemostasis of punctured blood vessels using high-intensity focused ultrasound. Ultrasound Med Biol 24:903–910
26. Wu F, Chen WZ, Bai J, Zou JZ, Wang ZL, Zhu H, Wang ZB (2002) Tumor vessel destruction resulting from high-intensity focused ultrasound in patients with solid malignancies. Ultrasound Med Biol 28:535–542
27. Vaezy S, Marti R, Mourad P, Crum L (1999) Hemostasis using high-intensity focused ultrasound. Eur J Ultrasound 9:79–87
28. Vaezy S, Martin R, Kaczkowski P, Keilman G, Goldman B, Yaziji H, Carter S, Caps M, Crum L (1999) Use of high-intensity focused ultrasound to control bleeding. J Vasc Surg 29:533–542
29. Vaezy S, Martin R, Crum L (2001) High-intensity focused ultrasound: a method of hemostasis. Echocardiography 18:309–315
30. Chen L, Rivens I, ter Haar G, Riddler S, Hill CR, Bensted JP (1993) Histological changes in rat liver tumours treated with high-intensity focused ultrasound. Ultrasound Med Biol 19:67–74

31. Köhrmann KU, Michel MS, Steidler A, Marlinghaus EH, Kraut O, Alken P (2002) Control parameters for high-intensity focused ultrasound (HIFU) for tissue ablation in the ex-vivo kidney (in German). Aktuel Urol 33:58–63

32. Wu F, Chen WZ, Bai J, Zou JZ, Wang ZL, Zhu H, Wang ZB (2001) Pathological changes in human malignant carcinoma treated with high-intensity focused ultrasound. Ultrasound Med Biol 27:1099–1106

33. Hynynen K, McDannold N, Vykhodtseva N, Jolesz FA (2001) Noninvasive MR imaging-guided focal opening of the blood-brain barrier in rabbits. Radiology 220: 640–646

34. Adams JB, Moore RG, Anderson JH, Strandberg JD, Marshall FF, Davoussi LR (1996) High-intensity focused ultrasound ablation of rabbit kidney tumors. J Endourol 10:71–75

35. Watkin NA, Morris SB, Rivens IH, ter Haar GR (1997) High-intensity focused ultrasound ablation of the kidney in a large animal model. J Endourol 11:191–196

36. Hill CR, ter Haar GR (1995) Review article: high-intensity focused ultrasound—potential for cancer treatment. Br J Radiol 68:1296–1303

37. Visioli AG, Rivens IH, ter Haar GR, Horwich A, Huddart RA, Moskovic E, Padhani A, Glees J (1999) Preliminary results of a phase I dose escalation clinical trial using focused ultrasound in the treatment of localised tumours. Eur J Ultrasound 9: 11–18

38. ter Haar G, Robertson G (1993) Tissue destruction with focused ultrasound in vivo. Eur Urol 23:8–11

39. Susani M, Madersbacher S, Kratzik C, Vingers L, Marberger M (1993) Morphology of tissue destruction induced by focused ultrasound. Eur Urol 23(Suppl 1):34–38

40. Köhrmann KU, Michel MS, Back W, Alken P (2000) Contactless tissue ablation in the kidney and prostate by high-intensity focused ultrasound (abstract). BJU Int 86(Suppl):207.

41. Köhrmann K, Michel M, Back W (2000) Non-invasive thermoablation in the kidney: first results of the clinical feasibility study. J Endourol 14(Suppl 1):A34

42. Chapelon JY, Margonari J, Theillere Y, Gorry F, Vernier F, Blanc E, Gelet A (1992) Effects of high-energy focused ultrasound on kidney tissue in the rat and the dog. Eur Urol 22:147–152

43. Averch TD, Adams JB, Anderson JH (1996) Transcutaneous ablation of rabbit tumors utilizing high-intensity focused ultrasound (abstract). J Urol 155:932

44. Daum DR, Smith NB, King R, Hynynen K (1999) In vivo demonstration of non-invasive thermal surgery of the liver and kidney using an ultrasonic phased array. Ultrasound Med Biol 25:1087–1098

45. Paterson RF, Barret E, Siqueira TM Jr, Gardner TA, Tavakkoli J, Rao VV, Sanghvi NT, Cheng L, Shalhav AL (2003) Laparoscopic partial kidney ablation with high-intensity focused ultrasound. J Urol 169:347–351

46. Häcker A, Michel MS, Knoll T, Marlinghaus E, Alken P, Köhrmann KU (2002) Non-invasive tissue ablation of kidney tumors by high-intensity focused ultrasound. J Urol 169:673

47. Chapelon JY, Margonari J, Vernier F, Gorry F, Ecochard R, Gelet A (1992) In vivo effects of high-intensity ultrasound on prostatic adenocarcinoma Dunning R3327. Cancer Res 52:6353–6357

98   A. Häcker et al.

48. Oosterhof GO, Cornel EB, Smits GA, Debruyne FM, Schalken JA (1997) Influence of high-intensity focused ultrasound on the development of metastases. Eur Urol 32:91–95
49. Gill IS, Novick AC, Meraney AM, Chen RN, Hobart MG, Sung GT, Hale J, Schweizer DK, Remer EM (2000) Laparoscopic renal cryoablation in 32 patients. Urology 56:748–753
50. Gervais DA, McGovern FJ, Arellano RS, McDougal WS, Mueller PR (2003) Renal cell carcinoma: clinical experience and technical success with radio-frequency ablation of 42 tumors. Radiology 226:417–424
51. Dechet CB, Zincke H, Sebo TJ, King BF, LeRoy AJ, Farrow GM, Blute ML (2003) Prospective analysis of computerized tomography and needle biopsy with permanent sectioning to determine the nature of solid renal masses in adults. J Urol 169:71–74
52. Rukstalis DB, Khorsandi M, Garcia FU, Hoenig DM, Cohen JK (2001) Clinical experience with open renal cryoablation. Urology 57:34–39
53. Rowland IJ, Rivens I, Chen L, Lebozer CH, Collins DJ, ter Haar GR, Leach MO (1997) MRI study of hepatic tumours following high-intensity focused ultrasound surgery. Br J Radiol 70:144–153

High-Intensity Focused Ultrasound (HIFU) for the Treatment of Localized Prostate Cancer

Toyoaki Uchida, Hiroshi Ohkusa, Hideyuki Yamashita, and Yoshihiro Nagata

Summary. We evaluated 85 patients with localized prostate cancer treated with high-intensity focused ultrasound (HIFU) for biochemical disease-free rate, safety, morbidity, and predictors of biochemical outcome. A total of 85 patients underwent HIFU with the use of Sonablate and with at least 12 months of follow-up. The median age was 70 years (range, 54 to 86 years), and the median preoperative prostate-specific antigen (PSA) level was 10.9 ng/ml (range, 3.39 to 89.6). The median length of follow-up was 20 months (range, 6 to 56). Biochemical failure was defined according to the criteria recommended by the American Society for Therapeutic Radiology and Oncology Consensus Panel. Biochemical failure developed in 27% (23/85) of the patients. The biochemical disease-free survival rates at 3 years for patients with pretreatment PSA less than 10 ng/ml, 10.01 to 20.0 ng/ml, 20.01 to 30.0 ng/ml, and more than 30.0 ng/ml were 97%, 75%, 33%, and 0%, respectively. Final follow-up sextant biopsies showed 91% (77/85) of the patients to be cancer free. Fifteen patients (18%) developed a urethral stricture, 3 patients (4%) underwent transurethral resection of the prostate for prolonged urinary retention or urethral stricture, 2 patients (2%) developed epididymitis, and 1 patient (1%) developed a rectourethral fistula. Twenty-eight percent (18/25) of the patients complained of postoperative erectile dysfunction. Accordint to multivariate analysis, preoperative PSA ($P < 0.0001$) and Gleason score ($P = 0.0466$) were significant independent predictors of time to biochemical recurrence. In conclusion, HIFU therapy appears to be a safe and efficacious minimally invasive therapy for patients with localized prostate cancer, especially those with a pretreatment PSA level less than 20 ng/ml.

Keywords. Localized prostate cancer, Minimally invasive therapy, High-intensity focused ultrasound

Department of Urology, Tokai University Hachioji Hospital, 1838 Ishikawa-machi, Hachioji, Tokyo 192-0032, Japan

Introduction

Prostate cancer is the leading malignancy in men and the second leading cause of death due to cancer in the United States [1]. In recent years, the rate of prostate cancer in Japanese males has also been increasing. In 1999 the death rate from prostate cancer in Japan increased from 4.5 to 11.4 per 100,000 men [2]. Prostate cancer is treated in various ways, depending on the severity of the condition, age of the patient, staging, Gleason score, and serum prostate-specific antigen (PSA) level. Despite excellent 5- to 10-year survival rates after radical prostatectomy for organ-confined disease, surgery is associated with significant morbidity, such as blood loss with transfusion-related complications, impotence in 30% to 70% of cases, and stress incontinence in up to 10% of patients [3–7]. In addition, surgical intervention is not typically considered for patients whose life expectancy is less than 10 years. Although the immediate complication rate is lower with radiation therapy, impotence, incontinence, radiation proctitis, and cystitis are frequent late sequelae [8, 9]. Recently, a number of alternative minimally invasive treatments have been developed to treat localized prostate cancer. Brachytherapy, cryosurgical ablation of the prostate, three-dimensional conformal radiotherapy (3D-CRT), intensity-modulated external beam radiotherapy (IMRT), and laparoscopic radical prostatectomy have been applied, but a definitive cure cannot always be achieved, and generally the treatment cannot be repeated in cases of local recurrence [10–14]. Since 1999, we have been treating localized prostate cancer with transrectal high-intensity focused ultrasound (HIFU) [15, 16]. HIFU delivers intense ultrasound energy, with consequent heat destruction of tissue at a specific focal distance from the probe without damage to tissue in the path of the ultrasound beam. We report herein our clinical experience treating 85 patients with stage T1c-2N0M0 localized prostate cancer by HIFU.

Materials and Methods

HIFU Equipment

For this study, we used a modified second- and third-generation device called the Sonablate 200 and 500 (Focus Surgery, Indianapolis, IN, USA) in 35 and 50 patients, respectively. A treatment module includes the ultrasound power generator, multiple transrectal probes of different focal depths, the probe positioning system, and a cooling system (Fig. 1). The transrectal HIFU probes use proprietary transducer technology with low-energy ultrasound (4MHz) for imaging of the prostate and for the delivery of high-energy ablative pulses (site intensity, 1300–2200 W/cm^2). The single piezoelectric crystal alternates between high-energy ablative (1–4sec) and low-energy (6–12sec) ultrasound for a total cycle of 7–16sec.

FIG. 1. The Sonablate
500 type device consists
of an operator's console,
imaging monitor,
transrectal probe, and an
automatic continuous
cooling system

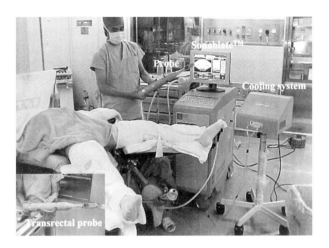

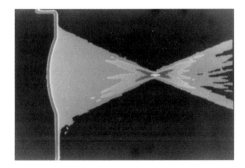

FIG. 2. High-intensity ultrasound was
focused on the specific lesion ($3 \times 3 \times 10$ mm)

Before the start of treatment, the operator uses longitudinal and transverse sonograms by imaging of the prostate and selects the prostate tissue volume to be ablated by a set of cursors on these images. The probe houses a computer-controlled positioning system that directs each ablative pulse to the targeted region of the prostate. Each discrete high-energy focused ultrasonic pulse ablates a volume of $2 \times 2 \times 10$ mm^3 in a single beam for 2.5-, 3.0-, 3.5-, 4.0-, and 4.5-cm focal length probes with Sonablate 200, and $3 \times 3 \times 10$ mm (Fig. 2) of tissue in a split beam for 3.0- and 4.0-cm focal length probes with Sonablate 500 [15–18]. For a single beam, the operation power density is set by the computer using the tissue depth measurements. In the split-beam mode, the total acoustic power is initially set at 24 and 37 W for 3.0- and 4.0-cm focal length probes, respectively. The individual focal lesion produces almost instantaneous coagulative necrosis of the tissue due to a temperature rise of 80° to 98°C in the focal zone [17, 18]. Under computer control, the ultrasound beam is steered mechanically to produce consecutive lesions in a manner such that all focal lesions overlap lat-

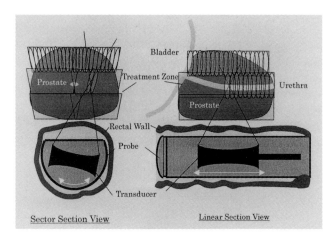

FIG. 3. The computer–controlled transducer ablates the entire prostate tissue. Focal lesions are overlapped in linear rows (*left*) at each of the lateral sector positions (*right*) to create a volume lesion

erally and longitudinally to ensure necrosis of the entire targeted prostate volume (Fig. 3). A semiautomatic or automatic cooling device is used during treatment to maintain a constant baseline temperature of less than 37° and 18°C in the transrectal probe that helps to prevent thermal injury of the rectal mucosa with the Sonablate 200 and 500, respectively.

HIFU Procedure

All patients were anesthetized by epidural or spinal anesthesia and were placed in the lithotomy position. A condom was placed over the probe, degassed water was used to inflate the condom, which was covered with ultrasound gel for close coupling of the ultrasound probe to the rectal wall, and the probe was inserted manually into the rectum. The probe was fixed in position by an articulating arm attached to the operating table. After selection of the treatment region of the prostate from the verumontanum to the bladder neck, the treatment was started. Transrectal probes with focal lengths of 2.5, 3.0, 3.5, 4.0, and 4.5 cm were used according to the size of the prostate, as determined by transrectal ultrasound (TRUS), with larger glands requiring longer focal lengths. The treatment continued layer by layer (10-mm thicknesses) from the apex to the base (Fig. 3). Usually, three successive target areas (anterior, mid-part, and base) were defined to treat the whole prostate (Fig. 4). After treatment had been completed, a transurethral balloon catheter, using a 14F or 16F Foley Balloon catheter, or percutaneous cystostomy was inserted into the bladder. Details of the HIFU techniques have been previously published [15, 16].

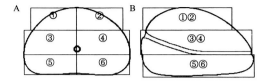

FIG. 4. Whole prostate including prostatic capsule was treated with 6 parts divided to right and left sides of anterior, mid and base-part of the prostate

Patient Recruitment

As a rule, the inclusion criteria for treatment were patients with stage T1c-2N0M0 localized prostate cancer and prostate volumes less than 50 ml. Patients with anal stricture were excluded from the study. All patients were fully informed of the details of this treatment and provided written consent preoperatively.

Between January 1999 and October 2002, 85 patients with clinically localized prostate cancer were treated with HIFU. Before undergoing HIFU, all patients underwent initial examination, including digital rectal examination. Pretreatment evaluation included history, physical examination (including digital rectal examination), initial PSA, and Gleason score on needle biopsy of the prostate. Serum PSA was determined by radioimmunoassay (Tandem-R method), with a normal range of 4.0 ng/ml or less and a minimal detectable level of 0.008 ng/ml. All patients had a negative radionuclide bone scan and computerized tomography of the abdomen and pelvis confirming absence of metastatic disease. Tumors were staged using the TNM staging system [19]. The median patient age was 70 years (range, 54 to 86). The median PSA level was 10.90 ng/ml (range, 3.39 to 89.60). The TNM stage was T1c in 49 patients (58%), T2a in 27 patients (31%), and T2b in 9 patients (11%). All patients had a histological diagnosis of prostatic adenocarcinoma according to the Gleason grading system. The histologic grade was Gleason score 3 to 4 in 17 patients, 5 to 7 in 61 patients, and 8 to 9 in 7 patients. Neoadjuvant hormonal therapy was delivered in 37 patients. The mean and median follow-up period for all patients was 20.6 and 20.0 months (range, 6 to 56), respectively.

Clinical Follow-up and Definition of Outcome

Patient status and treatment-related complications were followed up by all available means, including periodic patient visits and self-administered questionnaires dealing with urinary continence and erectile function. Serum PSA was usually assayed every 1 to 6 months during follow-up. Postoperative prostate biopsy was performed in all patients at 6 months postoperatively. The American Society for Therapeutic Radiology and Oncology (ASTRO) Consensus Panel criterion for biochemical failure, i.e., three consecutive increases in posttreatment PSA after a nadir has been achieved, was used to define biochemical failure [20]. The time to biochemical failure was defined as midway between the posttreatment PSA nadir and the first of three consecutive PSA increases. Prostate needle biopsies were performed in all patients at 6 months postoperatively. All patients had at least three PSA determinations during follow-up. None of the patients received androgen deprivation after HIFU or other anticancer therapy before documentation of a biochemical failure.

Statistical Analysis

All statistical analyses were performed using commercially available software (StatView 5.0, Abacus Concepts, Berkeley, CA, USA). The chi-squared test assessed the correlation between preoperative and postoperative parameters. The distributions of biochemical disease-free survival rates were calculated according to the Kaplan-Meier method, and the log-rank test was used to compare curves for groups. Age, clinical stage, Gleason score, volume of the prostate, neoadjuvant hormone therapy, and pretreatment serum PSA was analyzed to estimate the prognostic relevance in a multivariate Cox proportional-hazards regression model. All p values less than 0.05 reflected statistically significant differences.

Results

Seventy-one patients were treated in one HIFU session, 13 patients in two sessions, and 1 patient in three sessions, for a total of 100 procedures in 85 patients (1.2 sessions per patient). The reasons for repeat HIFU treatments were as follows: six patients were retreated because of short on (2 sec) or long off (8 to 12 sec) intervals; four patients were retreated for residual tumor; two patients were hemilaterally treated on the right or left lobe of the prostate; two patients needed a repeat session to treat the whole prostate because of larger prostate size (37.9 and 50.6 ml); and one patient was retreated because of machine trouble. The median operating time and hospitalization was 150 min (range 30 to 356 min) and 4.0 days (range 3 to 20). A gradual reduction in prostate volume occurred in all patients. The gland size decreased from an initial volume of 25.6 mL (range 9.3–68.8 mL) to a final median volume of 12.5 mL (range 2.7 to 55.2) (p < 0.0001) in average 6.5 months (range, 3–23) interval.

Table 1 demonstrates the crude incidence of biochemical disease-free according to demographic and pretreatment characteristics. Totally, 73% (62/85 patients) showed a PSA disease-free-free survival (Fig. 5). Pretreatment PSA showed a statistically significant difference (p < 0.001) but clinical stage (p = 0.1233) and Gleason scores (p = 0.0759) were not significant difference. The 2-year biochemical disease-free survival rates for patients stage T1c, T2a and T2b were 76%, 72% and 42% (Fig. 6), respectively (p = 0.0831). The biochemical disease-free survival rate at 2 years for patients Gleason scores 2 to 4, 5 to 7 and 8 to10 were 94%, 65% and 57% (Fig. 7), respectively (p = 0.0538). In addition, the biochemical disease-free survival rates at 2 years for patients pretreatment

TABLE 1. Patient characteristics

Characteristics	All Pts
No. pts	85
Mean/median age (range)	70.3/70.0 (54–86)
Mean/median PSA (ng/ml)	10.90/16.07
Mean/median prostate volume (ml)	27.8/25.6
Pretreatment PSA (%):	
10 or less	36 (42)
10.1–20	31 (36)
20.1–30	9 (11)
Greater than 30	9 (11)
Clinical stage (%):	
T1c	49 (58)
T2a	27 (32)
T2b	9 (10)
Gleason score (%):	
2–4	17 (20)
5–7	61 (72)
8–10	7 (8)

H.M., 78 yo, Stage T2aN0M0

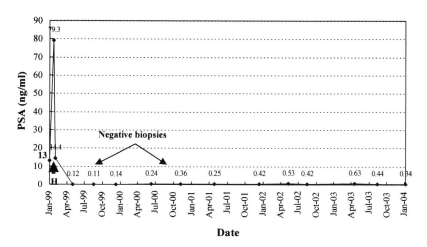

FIG. 5. Changes in serum PSA. Follow-up biopsies demonstrated intense coagulation necrosis at 2 months and extensive fibrotic tissue containing occasional atrophic glands without viable cancer cells at 6 and 10 months postoperatively. *H*, HIFU treatment

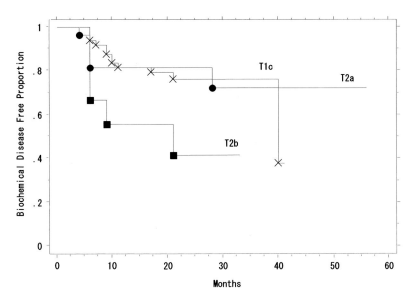

Fɪɢ. 6. Clinical stage and biochemical disease-free curve by Kaplan-Meier method

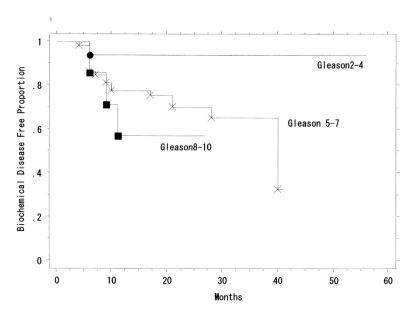

Fɪɢ. 7. Gleason score and biochemical disease-free curve by Kaplan-Meier method

PSA less than 10, 10.1 to 20, 20.1 to 30 and more than 30 ng/ml were 97%, 75%, 33% and 0% (Fig. 8), respectively (p < 0.0001).

In Cox regression analysis, preoperative PSA concentration (hazard ratio 1.059; p < 0.0001) and Gleason score (hazard ratio 1.440; p = 0.0466) demonstrated a statistically significant variables in these patients, but age, stages, prostatic volume, and neoadjuvant hormonal therapy were not statistically significant for prognosis (Table 2). Posttreatment prostate biopsies showed 91% (77/85) of the patients to be cancer free. The main pathological findings of prostate biopsy at 6 months after the procedure showed a coagulation necrosis and fibrosis.

Urinary symptoms such as frequency, urgency and difficulty urination were common during the first 2 months after HIFU treatment. The symptoms proved

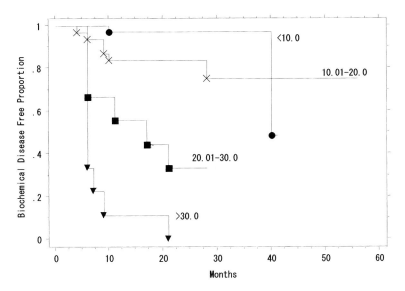

Fig. 8. Pretreatment PSA and biochemical disease-free curve by Kaplan-Meier method

Table 2. Cox proportional hazards analysis of patients predicting time to biochemical failure following HIFU

Parameters	Hazard Ratio	95%CI	P Value
Age	1.036	0.966–1.111	0.3257
Stage	0.610		
T1cN0M0	1.259	0.338–4.697	0.6827
T2aN0M0	0.722	0.152–3.437	0.9303
Gleason score	1.440	1.005–2.063	0.0466
Prostate volume	1.059	0.947–1.025	0.4659
Neoadjuvant therapy	0.680	0.224–2.057	0.4942
Preoperative PSA	1.059	1.036–1.082	<0.0001

to be transitory and were easily managed by medical treatment such as alpha-blockers or painkillers such as Voltaren suppository. Urethral catheter in all patients was removed 1 to 2 day postoperatively but catheter was re-indwelled in patients who could not urinate spontaneously and were tried to removal of catheter in every 1 to 2 weeks thereafter. The mean/median postoperative urinary catheterization time was 11/14 days (range 0–33 days). Final follow-up sextant biopsies showed 91% (77/85) of the patients to be cancer free. Fifteen (18%) patients developed a urethral stricture, 3 (4%) patients underwent transurethral resection of the prostate for prolonged urinary retention or ure-thral stricture, 2 (2%) and 1 (1%) patients developed epididymitis and a recto-urethral fistula. Twenty-eight % (18/25) patients complained postoperative erectile dysfunction. No incontinence was observed in follow-up.

Discussion

In 1995, Madersbacher et al. reported the effect of HIFU (using the old Sonab-late 200) in an experimental study of 10 cases of histologically demonstrated, hypoechoic and palpable, localized prostate cancer [18]. The organs were subse-quently removed in 2 weeks. The entire carcinoma had been ablated in two removed prostates, but in the other eight cases, a mean of 53% of the cancer tissue had been destroyed according to histopathological examination. In January 1999, we began HIFU treatment for localized prostate cancer using a modified Sonablate 200 device. Major improvements of our device included a reduction in the HIFU exposure cycle from 16 sec (4 on/12 off) to 9 sec (3 on/6 off), which reduced the treatment time by 44%; and the introduction of a novel transducer and electronics that splits a single ultrasound beam into multiple beams (termed "split beam") to cover a larger tissue volume per exposure. The single beam has a focal region of $2 \text{mm} \times 2 \text{mm} \times 10 \text{mm}$ (volume, 40mm^3), while the split beam focal region is $3 \text{mm} \times 3 \text{mm} \times 10 \text{mm}$ (volume, 90mm^3), which further reduces the treatment time by about 50% [15–18]. These developments dramatically shortened the treatment time for a 25-ml prostate gland from 6 h to 2 h.

In 1996, Gelet et al. reported a preliminary experience with HIFU using Ablatherm prototype 1.0 (EDAP-Technomed, Lyon, France) for treating local-ized prostate cancer [21]. They later summarized their clinical outcome, in which a complete response was obtained in 56% of the patients with no residual cancer and a PSA level less than 4 ng/ml. Biochemical failure (no residual cancer and a PSA level greater than 4 ng/ml), biochemical control (residual cancer and a PSA less than 4 ng/ml), and failure (residual cancer and a PSA level greater than 4.0 ng/ml) were noted in 6%, 18%, and 20% of patients, respectively. Several recent studies of HIFU therapy using Ablatherm devices have demonstrated a 73% to 56% rate of complete responses in patients with a negative biopsy and a PSA level less than 4.0 ng/ml [22–24]. In 1999, Beerlage et al. reported the results of 143 HIFU treatments using the Ablatherm prototype 1.0 and 1.1 in

111 patients with clinical stage T1-3N0M0 prostate cancer and a PSA level less than 25 ng/ml. The first 65 treatments in 49 patients were performed selectively (i.e., a unilateral or bilateral treatment in one or two sessions was performed, depending on the findings from TRUS and biopsies); in the second 78 treatments in 62 patients, the whole prostate was treated. A complete response (defined as a PSA level less than 4.0 ng/ml and a negative biopsy) was achieved in 60% of the patients whose whole prostate was treated and in 25% of the selectively treated patients [23]. In our study, two patients who were treated selectively in the right lobe of the prostate for adenocarcinoma identified by a prostate biopsy showed a gradual elevation of PSA as well as viable cancer cells in the untreated lobe according to a postoperative prostate biopsy. A second HIFU treatment was then performed on the whole prostate, and the PSA level remained low with a negative biopsy result. Recently, many methods of imaging analysis have been used to detect prostate cancer, including TRUS, computed tomography (CT), endorectal coil magnetic resonance imaging (MRI), and multiple biopsies of the prostate under TRUS. However, prostate cancer is a multifocal disease, and it is not yet possible to determine the sites of microscopic focus of cancer cells by imaging analysis alone. Therefore, the whole prostate must be treated, as the results of our study and other studies corroborate.

In an ideal comparison to assess efficacy of various treatment options for localized prostate cancer would be standardized. However, inherent differences exist between surgery and radiation that must be reflected in how we assess success or failure. Many response criteria have been applied after radical prostatectomy or irradiation therapy, including brachytherapy. As an indication of the progression of cancer after radical prostatectomy, some have used the presence of a detectable level of PSA, others have used a single value greater than 0.4 or 0.5 ng/ml, and others have used two consecutive values of 0.2 ng/ml or greater [25]. However, these criteria are not suitable to determine the clinical effect on patients with HIFU. Because the prostate is not removed by HIFU treatment such as radiation therapy and cryosurgery of the prostate, the ASTRO criterion was applied in our series [20]. Gelet et al. reported the clinical results of HIFU treatment using stricter response criteria [26]. Their criteria for determining failure included any positive biopsy regardless of the PSA concentration or three successive elevations of PSA with a velocity of at least 0.75 ng/year in patients with negative biopsy results. They reported that 62% of the patients exhibited no evidence of disease progression 60 months after HIFU. When we summarize our clinical outcome by the ASTRO criteria, 73% of the patients were biochemically disease free in our study. In particular, 97% and 75% of the patients whose PSA levels were less than 10.0 ng/ml and 10.01 to 20.0 ng/ml, respectively, were biochemically disease free. The clinical outcome in our series of patients with preoperative PSA levels less than 20 ng/ml were comparable to the outcome of patients treated with radical prostatectomy [5–7].

A disadvantage of HIFU treatment of localized prostate cancer is that there is a limit to the volume of the prostate gland that can be treated. The maximum volume that can be treated depends on the focal length of the transrectal probe.

In our experience, prostates with a volume greater than 50 ml cannot be treated with the present HIFU device, even with the use of a 4.5-cm focal length probe. It is necessary to develop a probe with a longer focal length probe to treat prostates more than 50 ml in volume. Neoadjuvant androgen deprivation therapy may be useful in larger prostates, especially since reduction of the target volume may increase the efficacy of the HIFU treatment. In addition, patients with intraprostatic large calcifications are not suitable for HIFU, because the ultrasound beam is reflected by calcifications which may make a coagulation necrosis at unexpected lesion by reflected ultrasound. These limitations will be resolved by the further development of HIFU.

In our study, postoperative urinary retention for more than one day was noted in 80% of the patients who were required of catheterization with balloon catheter for 7.4 day in average. We have applied percutaneous cystostomy to prevent postoperative urinary retention in three patients, but these patients showed a longer urinary retention (mean, 39.0 days) than patients with balloon catheter (mean, 7.4 days). Intermittent self-catheterization, transient placement of prostatic stents, or postoperative transurethral resection of the prostate (TURP) might solve this problem. A rectourethral fistula occurred in one patient after a second HIFU treatment. More precise HIFU power control is needed at repeat treatments. At present, a continuous cooling device is applied to keep the rectal mucosa at a temperature below 20°C during the procedure. No rectourethral fistula was noted in any patients after use of the automatic cooling system. Postoperative urethral strictures near the verumontanum in the prostatic urethra occurred in 18% of patients and were treated by internal urethrotomy and/or periodic dilation with metal sounds. Performance of TURP after HIFU treatment may be useful to prevent postoperative urethral stricture or urinary retention.

Whether to perform radical prostatectomy is controversial because of its effects on sexual function. Prevention of postoperative impotence depends on preservation of neurovascular bundles that sometimes include invasive tumor. In our study, 28% of the patients exhibited erectile dysfunction after HIFU therapy. We consider that this rate is low in comparison with the rate after radical prostatectomy [3–5]. The color Doppler ultrasound system may reduce the rate of erectile dysfunction by identifying neurovascular bundles more accurately. Further experience is required to address this important problem.

Conclusion

For many reasons, transrectal HIFU appears highly attractive as a minimally invasive treatment for localized prostate cancer. HIFU treatment requires no incision or puncture, it is bloodless, it can be performed on an outpatient basis, and repeatable added even though patients with local recurrence have already been treated with radiation therapy. In addition, the option of HIFU may be more attractive to the patient who wants to avoid postoperative incontinence and erectile dysfunction for his quality of life. The small number of patients and the relatively short follow-up period in our series limit our ability to draw any definitive conclusions. We believe that the data we present here suggest that HIFU may be a useful treatment option for patients with localized prostate cancer. Our goal to be able to treat patients with localized prostate cancer by HIFU within one hour in an outpatient clinic under local anesthesia.

Acknowledgments. The authors express their appreciation to Y. Shimazaki, S. Kagosaki, K. Yamashita, K. Takai, and N. T. Sanghvi for their technical assistance.

References

1. Landis SH, Murray T, Bolden S, Wingo PA (1999) Cancer statistics, 1999. CA Cancer J Clin 49:8–31
2. Statistics and Information Department, Minister's Secretariat, Ministry of Health and Welfare, Health and Welfare Statistics Association (2000) Statistical Abstract on Health and Welfare in Japan 2000. Health and Welfare Statistics Association, Tokyo, p 55
3. Merrill RM, Morris MK (2002) Prevalence-corrected prostate cancer incidence and trends. Am J Epidemiol 155:148–152
4. Arai Y, Egawa S, Tobisu K, Sagiyama K, Sumiyoshi Y, Hashine K, Kawakita M, Matsuda T, Matsumoto K, Fujimoto H, Okada T, Kakehi Y, Terachi T, Ogawa O (2000) Radical retropubic prostatectomy: time trends, morbidity and mortality in Japan. BJU Int 85:287–294
5. Amling CL, Blute ML, Bergstralh EJ, Seay TM, Slezak J, Zincke H (2000) Long-term hazard of progression after radical prostatectomy for clinically localized prostate cancer: continued risk of biochemical failure after 5 years. J Urol 164:101–105
6. Han M, Walsh PC, Partin AW, Rodriguez R (2000) Ability of the 1992–1997 American Joint Committee on Cancer Staging for Prostate Cancer to predict progression-free survival after radical prostatectomy for stage T2 disease. J Urol 164:89–92
7. Hull GW, Rabbani F, Abbas F, Wheeler TM, Kattan MW, Scardino PT (2002) Cancer control with radical prostatectomy alone in 1000 consecutive patients. J Urol 167:528–534
8. Rosser CJ, Levy LB, Kuban DA, Chichakli R, Pollack A, Lee A, Pisters LL (2003) Hazard rates of disease progression after external beam radiotherapy for clinically localized carcinoma of the prostate. J Urol 169:2160–2165
9. Zietman AL, Chung CS, Coen JJ, Shipley WU (2004) 10-year outcome for men with localized prostate cancer treated with external radiation therapy: results of a cohort study. J Urol 171:210–214

10. Vicini FA, Kini VR, Edmundson G, Gustafson GS, Stromberg J, Martinez A (1999) A comprehensive review of prostate cancer brachytherapy: defining an optional technique. Int J Radiat Oncol Biol Phys 44:483–491

11. Han K-R, Cohen JK, Miller RJ, Pantuck AJ, Freitas DG, Cuevas CA, Kim HL, Lugg J, Childs SJ, Shuman B, Jayson MA, Shore ND, Moore Y, Zisman A, Lee JY, Ugarte R, Mynderse LA, Wilson TM, Sweat SD, Zincke H, Belldegran AS (2003) Treatment of organ confined prostate cancer with third generation cryosurgery: preliminary multicenter experience. J Urol 170:1126–1130

12. Zelefsky MJ, Wallner KE, Ling CC, Raben A, Hollister T, Wolfe T, Grann A, Gaudin P, Fuks Z, Leibel SA (1999) Comparison of the 5-year outcome and morbidity of three-dimensional conformal radiotherapy versus transperineal permanent iodine-125 implantation for early stage prostate cancer. J Clin Oncol 17:517–522

13. Beerlage HP, Thuroff S, Madersbacher S, Zlotta AR, Aus G, de Reijke TM, de la Rosette JJMCH (2000) Current status of minimally invasive treatment options for localized prostate carcinoma. Eur Urol 37:2–13

14. Guillonneau B, el-Fettouh H, Baumert H, Cathelineau X, Doublet JD, Fromont G, Vallancien G (2003) Laparoscopic radical prostatectomy: oncological evaluation after 1000 cases a Montsouris Institute. J Urol 169:1261–1266

15. Uchida T, Sanghvi NT, Gardner TA, Koch MO, Ishii D, Minei S, Satoh, T, Hyodo T, Irie A, Baba S (2000) Transrectal high-intensity focused ultrasound for treatment of patients with stage T1b-2N0M0 localized prostate cancer: a preliminary report. Urology 59:394–399

16. Uchida T, Tsumura H, Yamashita H, Katsuta M, Ishii D, Satoh T, Ohkawa A, Hyodo T, Sanghvi NT (2003) Transrectal high-intensity focused ultrasound for treatment of patients with stage T1b-2N0M0 localized prostate cancer: a preliminary report. Jpn J Endourol ESWL 16:108–114

17. Wu JSY, Sanghvi NT, Phillips MH, Kuznetsov M, Foster RS, Bihrle R, Gardner TA, Umemura SI (1999) Experimental studies of using of split beam transducer for prostate cancer therapy in comparison to single beam transducer. 1999 IEEE Ultrasonics Symposium Proceedings 2:1443–1446

18. Madersbacher S, Pedevilla M, Vingers L, Susani M, Merberger M (1995) Effect of high-intensity focused ultrasound on human prostate cancer in vivo. Cancer Res 55:3346–3351

19. International Union Against Cancer (1997) TNM classification of malignant tumors, Ed. by Sobin LH and Witteikind CH, pp 170–173. Wiley and Sons, New York

20. Consensus statement (1997) Guidelines for PSA following radiation therapy. American Society for Therapeutic Radiology and Oncology Consensus Panel. Int J Radiat Oncol Biol Phys 37:1035–1041

21. Gelet A, Chaperon JY, Bouvier R, Souchon R, Pangaud C, Abdelrahim AF, Cathignol D, Dubernnard JM (1996) Treatment of prostate cancer with transrectal focused ultrasound: early clinical experience. Eur Urol 29:174–183

22. Gelet A, Chaperon JY, Bouvier R, Pagnaud C, Lasne Y (1999) Local control of prostate cancer by transrectal high intensity focused ultrasound therapy: preliminary report. J Urol 161:156–162

23. Beerlage HP, Thüroff S, Debruyne FMJ, Chaussy C, de la Rosette JJMCH (1999) Transrectal high-intensity focused ultrasound using the Ablatherm device in the treatment of localized prostate carcinoma. Urology 54:273–277

24. Chaussy CG, Thüroff S (2000) High-intensity focused ultrasound in localized prostate cancer. J Endourol 14:293–299
25. Moul JW (2000) Prostate specific antigen only progression of prostate cancer. J Urol 163:1632–1642
26. Gelet A, Chapelon JY, Bouvier R, Rouviere O, Lasne Y, Lyonnet D, Dubernard JM (2000) Transrectal high-intensity focused ultrasound: minimally invasive therapy of localized prostate cancer. J Endourol 14:519–528

Renal Cryoablation

KEN NAKAGAWA and MASARU MURAI

Summary. With the widespread use of imaging modalities, the majority of renal tumors are incidentally detected as small masses. Although these small tumors have been traditionally treated with radical nephrectomy, partial nephrectomy has recently become accepted as a nephron-sparing surgery (NSS). In the stream of minimally invasive therapy (MIT), laparoscopic partial nephrectomy has been established, but some problems, such as bleeding, urine leakage, and A-V shunt, still remain after the operation. Currently, energy ablation therapies with some approaches are evaluated to manage small renal-cell carcinomas. Ablation therapy, combined with MIT and NSS, is a potential new-generation therapy. Among the various ablation therapies, cryosurgery is the most notable for its high local control rates in initial clinical studies. In this review, the principles of cryoablation and the initial clinical results of renal cryoablation are assessed and our clinical experience with renal cryoablation are reported. Renal cryoablation appears to be a safe and effective minimally invasive alternative for the treatment of small renal masses. However, careful selection of patients with lesions that are less than 3 cm in diameter and close monitoring of the iceball are necessary for successful treatment, and long follow-up is also mandatory for final establishment.

Keywords. Cryoablation, Small renal-cell carcinoma, Laparoscopic surgery, Nephron-sparing surgery, Minimally invasive therapy

Introduction

With the widespread use of imaging modalities, the majority of renal tumors are incidentally detected as small masses [1]. They are known to have low biologic malignant activity [2]. Although these small tumors have traditionally been

Department of Urology, Keio University School of Medicine, 35 Shinanomachi, Shinjuku-ku, Tokyo 160-8582, Japan

treated with radical nephrectomy, partial nephrectomy has recently become accepted as a nephron-sparing surgery (NSS). In the treatment of small (<4 cm) renal-cell carcinomas (RCCs), NSS is equally effective as radical nephrectomy [3]. However, its open procedure is not associated with a decrease in postoperative suffering or hospital stay. Meanwhile, laparoscopic surgery has been developed, and laparoscopic radical nephrectomy has offered advantages with regard to morbidity and convalescence. In the stream of minimally invasive therapy (MIT), laparoscopic partial nephrectomy has been established, but some problems, such as bleeding, urine leakage, and A-V shunt, still remain after the operation. Finally, energy ablation therapies with some approaches are evaluated to manage small RCCs. Ablation therapy, combined with MIT and NSS, is a potential new-generation therapy. The energy ablation therapies include cryoablation (or cryosurgery), radiofrequency ablation, and microwave ablation; cryosurgery is the most notable for its high local control rates in initial clinical studies.

Historical Background

Cryosurgery is the use of subzero temperatures for in situ tissue destruction [4]. In the middle of the 19th century, low temperature was produced by crushed ice and salt solutions. Using this method, Arnott reduced the size of tumors and ameliorated pain in patients with advanced breast and cervical cancer [5]. However, despite the introduction of solidified carbon dioxide and liquid oxygen, cryosurgery was limited to topical application during the early 1900s.

During the 1960s, Cooper introduced a modern, automated cryosurgical apparatus with liquid nitrogen in neurosurgery. The Joule-Thomson effect describes the rapid cooling that results from the rapid phase change of highly compressed liquid nitrogen expanding through a restricted orifice to a gaseous state [6]. This led to renewed interest in cryosurgery and its possible applications. The biology of cryosurgery has been known for decades, and intraoperative ultrasound imaging has permitted recent clinical applications for the treatment of small renal tumors. Percutaneous [7] and open [8, 9] surgical approaches have been used to deliver cryotherapy. Recent studies have focused on minimally invasive therapy using cryosurgery as NSS [10–12].

Principles of Cryosurgery

Tissue destruction from cryosurgery is typically described in two phases: freezing and thawing. A liquid nitrogen or liquid argon system is used during the freeze part of the treatment cycle in modern cryosurgery, whereas the thaw portion is usually carried out with helium gas. The freezing phase is performed

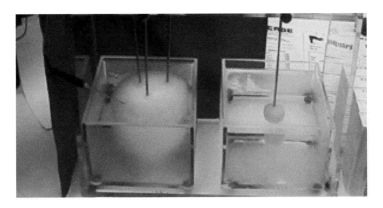

FIG. 1. Iceball

rapidly with the generation of an iceball with a core temperature of –196°C (Fig. 1). Freezing creates cell death by several mechanisms. Subfreezing conditions cause formation of intracellular ice crystals, which creates a hyperosmolar environment. This environment in turn causes cell dehydration and shrinkage, enzyme denaturation, and dysfunction of the cytoskeleton and membrane. Additional damage may be produced by microvascular thrombosis and cellular anoxia. Rapid freezing followed by gradual thawing, known as a double freeze-thaw cycle, is used to maximize these effects [13].

The process of cryoablation is dependent on the temperature of the cryoprobe, the area of contact of the freezing surface, and the thermal conductivity of the tissue [14]. Differences between tissue resistances to freezing are also dependent on the distance from large vessels. This phenomenon is known as the heat sink effect. Theoretically, this heat sink or thermal conduction can affect the rate of cooling and the size of the cryoablation and prolong the time needed to reach any given temperature. Renal artery clamping has been attempted to increase the ablation effect but has not proved valuable.

The most important parameter affecting tissue necrosis within the cryolesion is temperature. An experiment in a porcine model using thermocouples indicated that a temperature of –19.4°C must be achieved to ensure completely homogeneous necrosis [15]. It also demonstrated uniform ablation of tissue at a distance of 16 mm or less from the cryoprobe, whereas all samples taken from a distance >21 mm from the cryoprobe were viable. The area of necrosis produced by the cryoprobe is visually approximated as the iceball, but temperatures higher than –20°C exist at its periphery. Campbell and associates [16] achieved a temperature of –20°C at 3.1 mm behind the leading edge of the iceball in all 10 animals tested, suggesting extension of the iceball at least this distance beyond the edge of the tumor being treated to ensure adequate cooling.

Intraoperative Monitoring

Because of its nature as an NSS, destruction of tumor tissue must be complete while minimizing damage to the surrounding healthy parenchyma. Expansion of the iceball into other adjacent organs, such as the colon, is also a concern. To achieve NSS, real-time monitoring of the cryolesion is very important. Open and laparoscopic cryosurgery permit monitoring by direct observation, ultrasonography, and thermocouples. Direct observation of the iceball during the freeze-thaw cycle is the simplest monitoring. The periphery of the iceball can be estimated by the change in tissue appearance, as well as the formation of ice crystals on the surface of the frozen tissue (Fig. 2). Intraoperative ultrasonography accurately delineates tumor size, cryoprobe placement, and depth of freezing [17]. An anechoic, avascular sphere with an advancing, hyperechoic rim characterizes the real-time intraoperative ultrasound image of renal cryolesions (Fig. 3) [18]. However, ultrasound monitoring of the complete iceball is difficult because the frozen tissue shows an acoustic shadow, resulting in visibility of only the near edge of the iceball. Only the placement of thermocouples can allow an accurate predictor of tissue destruction as tissue temperature. In magnetic resonance imaging (MRI)- or computed tomographic (CT)-guided cryoablation, each axial imaging becomes the good monitoring modality. With MRI, the short T_2 of ice leaves the frozen region black against a background of normal tissue [18]. CT imaging detects a sharply defined margin around frozen tissue, with a decrease of attenuation of approximately 30 Hounsfield unit (HU) in frozen tissue compared with adjacent unfrozen tissue [19].

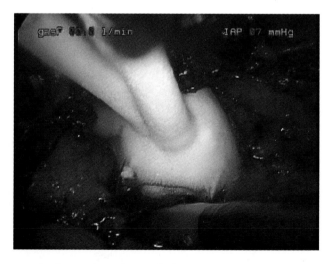

FIG. 2. Laparoscopic observation of a cryolesion

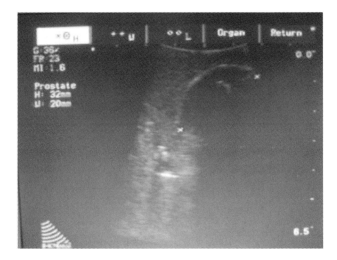

FIG. 3. Iceball on ultrasonography. An acoustic shadow is recognized behind the iceball

Postoperative Changes

Acute histological changes include ill-defined cell borders, epithelial exfoliation, vesicular nuclei, hemorrhagic glomeruli with capillary fibrin deposition, and intramural hemorrhage in large vessels [20]. Later changes are indicative of coagulation necrosis, which is eventually replaced by fibrotic scarring.

For postoperative follow-up, gadolinium-enhanced MRI has been used [18]. On postoperative day 1, MRI routinely shows a concentric, nonenhancing defect in the ablated area. All lesions are isointense on T_1-weighted images and hypointense on T_2-weighted images. About half of the lesions demonstrate an increase in signal intensity on both T_1- and T_2-weighted images, but no enhancement. Serial examinations reveal spontaneous contraction and shrinkage of the lesion with a decrease in size of 8%, 23%, 40%, and 48% at 1, 2, 3, and 6 months, respectively.

Approaches and Clinical Studies

Cryoablation has been performed using the open, percutaneous, or laparoscopic approach since Uchida et al. reported the first percutaneous renal cryoablation [7]. They performed cryoablation in two patients with advanced RCC under general anesthesia and ultrasound guidance. The largest published human series to date is that of laparoscopic cryoablation by Gill et al. [18]. They have performed over 34 renal cryoablations in 32 patients. All lesions were small (<4 cm), peripheral, exophytic, and solid. Anteriorly located tumors were approached transperitoneally, and posterior tumors were approached retroperitoneally. At six-month follow-up, all evaluated cases had negative findings on MRI and needle biopsy. However, in the further results one case was reported with a local recurrence. Postoperative renal function at 24h was unchanged in this study. There was no evidence of urine leakage. One patient was noted to have a peri-renal hematoma. Rukstalis et al. treated 29 patients with an open procedure [21]. At a mean follow-up of 16 months, 91.3% of patients had a complete response according to MRI, and there was one biopsy-proved local recurrence. There were more complications in the open group, including ensuing renal failure in three patients, one conversion to nephrectomy, and one persistent RCC on short-term postprocedural imaging. Shingleton and Sewell reported a percutaneous series under general anesthesia [12]. At a mean follow-up of 9.1 months, there was no evidence of tumor recurrence, although one patient required retreatment due to continuing residual enhancement in the treated area. A wound abscess requir-ing drainage developed in one patient. It appears that all three approaches offer similar results as long as the tumor can be successfully localized and the probe inserted safely.

Clinical Experience

As stated above, renal cryoablation has been proposed as a clinically viable option for the treatment of small renal tumors. Here, we introduce our clinical experiences of renal cryoablation.

Materials and Methods

Patient

From December 2002 to March 2004, 14 patients underwent renal cryoablation therapy at Keio university hospital (Table 1). All patients were candidates for partial nephrectomy for renal malignancies (14 patients with RCC, 1 with metastatic sarcoma) and the renal tumors were less than 4 cm in diameter (mean, 2.2 ± 0.6 cm; range, 1.5–4.0 cm). The mean age of the patients was 57.1 ± 12.0 years (range, 41–81 years). Three of the patients were treated with chemotherapy for other malignancies, two had liver cirrhosis, and two received anticoagulant therapy for ischemic diseases. One patient had bilateral lesions. Thirteen patients were treated with laparoscopic cryoablation (transperitoneal or retroperitoneal approaches), and one was treated with CT-guided percutaneous cryoablation.

Technique

The laparoscopic approach used was dependent on the location of the tumor. Posterior, lateral, and lower anterolateral tumors were approached retroperi-toneally; anterior and upper anterolateral tumors were approached transperi-toneally. Three- or four-port procedures were employed with the patient in the lateral position under general anesthesia. Briefly, the operative steps included

TABLE 1. Patient characteristics

Case	Age (years)	Sex	Side	Tumor size (cm)	Approach	Background
1	49	F	L	4.0	Retro	Postchemotherapy
2	60	M	R	2.3	Laparo	
3	53	M	R	2.4	Retro	Liver cirrhosis
4	60	M	R	1.6	Retro	Liver cirrhosis
5	41	M	L	3.5	Retro	
6	56	M	L	1.6	Retro	Angina
7	50	M	L	2.2	Retro	
8	46	F	L	2.3	Retro	Postchemotherapy
9	67	M	L	1.5	Retro	Postchemotherapy
10	45	M	R	2.1	Retro	
11	81	M	R	1.7	Percutaneous (CT)	Angina
12	56	M	L	2.5	Retro	
13	58	M	L	2.0	Retro	
14	54	M	L	2.0	Retro	

Mean 57.1 ± 12.0   2.2 ± 0.6

L, left; R, right; Retro, retroperitoneally; Laparo, laparoscopically; CT, computed-tomography-guided

mobilization of the kidney within Gerota's fascia; excision of the overlying perirenal fat for histologic examination; imaging of the tumor with a laparoscopic ultrasound probe; and laparoscopic needle biopsy of the tumor, followed by puncture renal cryoablation under laparoscopic and ultrasonographic guidance. A double freeze-thaw cycle was performed with the aim of extending the iceball approximately 1 cm beyond the edge of the tumor or reaching the temperature of the thermocouple, which was placed beyond the periphery of a tumor, less than −20°C. Care was taken to keep the bowel, ureter, and other adjacent organs away from the iceball. The Cryocare Surgical System (Endocare, Irvine, CA, USA) (Fig. 4), an argon-helium-based system, was used for cryoablation. A 3-mm CryoProbe (Endocare) was placed for tumors less than 20 mm in diameter, and a 5-mm probe for tumors 20 to 30 mm in diameter. The use of multiple cryoprobes was considered for tumors over 30 mm in diameter. The puncture was filled up with Fibrin glue and/or Gelfoam after removal of the cryoprobe.

CT-guided percutaneous cryoablation was performed with the patient prone under local anesthesia (Fig. 5). A 3-mm cryoprobe was placed with its corresponding pinnacle introducer sheath.

Results

The lesions were treated successfully in all 14 patients. One patient (case 3) had urine leakage from the ureter 3 days after cryoablation and needed treatment with a ureteral catheter. There were no other intraoperative or perioperative complications. The mean operative time was 194 ± 32 min (range, 118–240 min), and the estimated blood loss was less than 50 ml (Table 2). The mean first freezing time was 11.5 ± 2.8 min (range, 7–17 min), and the second was 11.9 ± 3.3 min

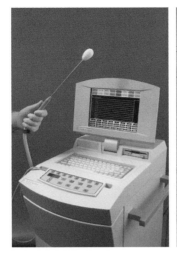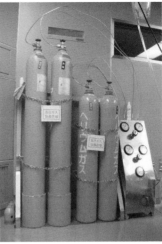

FIG. 4. Cryocare Surgical System (Endocare, Irvine, CA, USA)

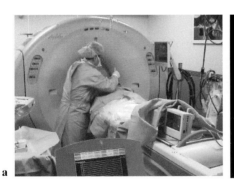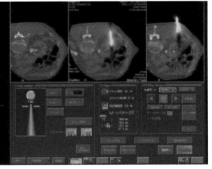

a   b

FIG. 5. Computed tomography (CT)-guided percutaneous cryoablation. **a** Outside appearance. **b** CT imaging

(range, 5–20 min). The lowest temperature of the thermocouple placed periphery was −29.8°C (range, −12.0 to −64.1°C). The average use of analgesics was 0.6 ± 1.0 times (range, 0–3) (Table 3). The mean length of return to normal activity was 4.3 ± 0.7 days (range, 3–6 days), except for the one patient with urine leakage. No patients needed readmission to the hospital after discharge. The mean serum creatinine level was 0.9 ± 0.3, 0.8 ± 0.4, and 0.9 ± 0.3 mg/dl on day −1, day 1, and day 3, respectively (Fig. 6). CT imaging on day 2 did not show any complicated findings, including hemorrhage, and all the areas of cryoablation were not enhanced (Fig. 7).

Thirteen of the 14 patients did not have any findings of recurrence or metastasis on enhanced CT during follow-up (mean, 10.1 ± 5.2 months; range, 1–16

TABLE 2. Intraoperative data

Case	Operative time (min)	Probe (mm)	Thermocouple (°C)	Freeze 1 (min)	Freeze 2 (min)
1	205	5 × 2	−40.2	10	11
2	205	5 × 1	−32.0	10	10
3	182	5 × 1	−12.0	13	12
4	170	3 × 1	−21.6	10	10
5	209	5 × 1	−23.7	15	12
6	240	3 × 1	−50.7	7	5
7	181	5 × 1	−34.9	10	12
8	124	5 × 1	−30.7	12	13
9	210	5 × 1	−26.3	8	20
10	215	5 × 1	−31.0	12	10
11[a]	240	3 × 1		15	15
12	118	5 × 1	−64.1	10	12
13	208	5 × 1	−27.6	17	10
14	165	5 × 1	−12.8	12	14
Mean,	194 ± 32		−29.8	11.5 ± 2.8	11.9 ± 3.3

[a] Case 11 underwent a CT-guided percutaneous procedure

TABLE 3. Postoperative data

Case	No. of analgesics	Return to normal activity (days)	Complications	Follow-up (mo)	Recurrence
1	1	4	—	16	—
2	3	5	—	16	—
3	0	5	—	15	—
4	1	4	—	15	—
5	2	9	Ureteral injury	13	Local
6	0	5	—	12	—
7	0	6	—	12	—
8	0	4	—	11	—
9	2	4	—	11	—
10	0	4	—	9	—
11[a]	0	3	—	5	—
12	0	4	—	4	—
13	0	4	—	2	—
14	0	4	—	1	—
Mean	0.6	4.8 ± 1.5		10.1 ± 5.2	

[a] Case 11 underwent a CT-guided percutaneous procedure

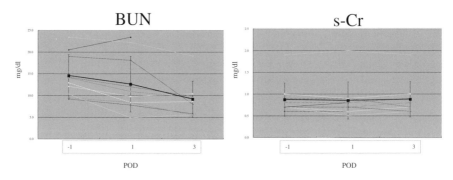

FIG. 6. Renal function. Cryoablation did not affect renal function. *BUN*, Blood urea nitrogen; *s-CR*, serum creatinine; *POD*, post operative day

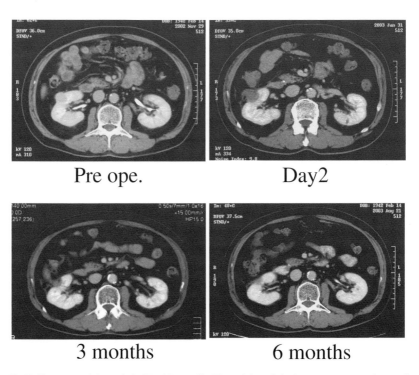

FIG. 7. Follow-up with serial CT (Case 2). The ablated lesion was not enhanced and became smaller on follow-up

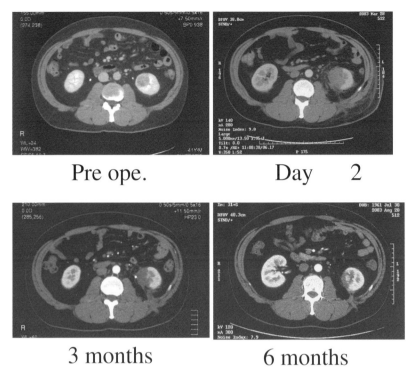

Pre ope.   Day   2

3 months   6 months

Fig. 8. Local recurrence in Case 5. An enhanced lesion was recognized in the ablated area after 3 months of follow-up

months), and renal function was well preserved over the period. Seven patients underwent needle biopsy 6 months after cryoablation, and there were no findings of malignancy. However, one patient, who had a 35-mm tumor ablated with one 5-mm probe, was diagnosed as having a local recurrence on CT after 3 months (Fig. 8), and he underwent laparoscopic radical nephrectomy 6 months after cryoablation.

Discussion

The laparoscopic approach provided superior operative exposure and good ultrasonographic exposure. We were able to achieve correct placement of the cryoprobe in laparoscopic cryoablation, and the results for tumors less than 3 cm in diameter were excellent during the follow-up. Cryoablation with multiple sticks for large tumors often made a crack in the tumor or normal renal parenchyma resulting from the iceball, although it did not lead to obvious troubles in our series. Therefore, at this stage, it may be preferable to limit treatment to single-stick cryoablation for small renal tumors (<3 cm). With this limitation, the correct placement of the probe in a laparoscopic operation is very important, because the area completely ablated with a single probe is strictly limited. Also, a laparoscopic approach is suitable to keep the adjacent organs away from the iceball. CT-guided or MRI-guided cryoablation would be available for smaller posterolateral tumors. It is our impression that it is somewhat difficult to supply a strict and safe placement of a probe for an anteromedial 3-cm tumor by the percutaneous approach.

When it is performed by an expert laparoscopic urologist, laparoscopic partial nephrectomy is a good treatment as an NSS and as an MIT. Nevertheless, we believe that laparoscopic cryoablation has advantages compared with partial nephrectomy: there is less blood loss; it does not involve renal hilar clamping and warm ischemia; it does not involve technically difficult suturing; it does not result in urine leaks; and it is effective in patients on anticoagulation. It offers advantages compared with partial nephrectomy in that it is easier to treat less exophytic tumors with this method. It also may reduce the possibility of hypertension caused by A-V fistula at the treated area.

Conclusion

Renal cryoablation appears to be a safe and effective minimally invasive alternative for the treatment of small renal masses. Careful selection of patients with lesions that are less than 3 cm in diameter and close monitoring of the iceball are necessary for successful treatment. Close and prolonged follow-up is also mandatory.

References

1. Smith SJ, Bosniak MA, Megibow AJ, Hulnick DH, Horii SC, Raghavendra BN (1989) Renal cell carcinoma: earlier discovery and increased detection. Radiology 170: 699–703
2. Bosniak MA, Brinbaum BA, Krinsky GA, Waisman J (1995) Small renal parenchymal neoplasms: further observations on growth. Radiology 197:589–597
3. Novic AC (1998) Nephron-sparing surgery for renal cell carcinoma. Br J Urol 82:321–324
4. Gage AA (1998) History of cryosurgery. Semin Surg Oncol 14:99–109
5. Arnott J (1850) Practical illustrations of remedial efficacy of a very low or anaesthetic temperature I: In cancer. Lancet 2:257–259
6. Baust J, Gage AA, Ma H, Zhang CM (1997) Minimally-invasive cryosurgery—technological advances. Cryobiology 34:373–384
7. Uchida M, Imaide Y, Sugimoto K, Vehara H, Watanabe H (1995) Percutaneous cryosurgery for renal tumors. Br J Urol 745:132–137
8. Delworth MG, Pisters LL, Fornage BD, von Eschenbach AC (1995) Cryotherapy for renal cell carcinoma and angiomyolipoma. J Urol 155:252–255

9. Rodriguez R, Chan DY, Bishoff JT, Chen RB, Kavoussi LR, Choti MA, Marshall FF (2000) Renal ablative cryosurgery in select patients with peripheral renal masses. Urology 55:25–30

10. Gill IS, Novic AC, Soble JJ, Sung GT, Remer EM, Hale J, O'Malley CM (1998) Laparoscopic renal cryoablation: initial clinical series. Urology 52:543–551

11. Johnson DB, Nakada SY (2000) Laparoscopic cryoablation for renal cell cancer. J Endourol 14:873–879

12. Shingleton WB, Sewell PE Jr (2001) Percutaneous renal tumor cryoablation with magnetic resonance imaging guidance. J Urol 165:773–776

13. Woolley ML, Schulsinger DA, Durand DB, Zeltser IS, Waltzer WC (2002) Effect of freezing parameters (freeze cycle and thaw process) on tissue destruction following renal cryoablation. J Endourol 16:519–522

14. Neel HB, Ketcham AS, Hammond WG (1971) Requistes for successful cryogenic surgery of cancer. Arch Surg 102:45–48

15. Chosy SG, Nakada SY, Lee FT Jr, Warner TF (1998) Monitoring renal cryosurgery: predictors of tissue necrosis in swine. J Urol 159:1370–1374

16. Campbell SC, Krishnamurthi G, Chow G, Hale J, Myles J, Novick AC (1998) Renal cryosurgery: experimental evaluation of treatment parameters. Urology 52:29–34

17. Zegel HG, Holland GA, Jennings SB, Chong WK, Cohen JK (1998) Intraoperative ultrasonographically guided cryoablation of renal masses: initial experience. J Ultrasound Med 17:571–576

18. Gill IS, Novic AC, Meraney AM, Chen RN, Hobart MG, Sung GT, Hale J, Schweizer DK, Remer EM (2000) Laparoscopic renal cryoablation in 32 patients. Urology 56:748–753

19. Passe GR, Wong STS, Roos MS, Rubinsky B (1995) MR imaging-guided control of cryosurgery. J Magn Reson Imaging 5:753–760

20. Saiken JC, McKinnon JG, Gray R (1996) CT for monitoring cryotherapy. Am J Roentgenol 166:853–855

21. Nakada SY, Lee FT Jr, Warner T, Chosy SG, Moon TD (1998) Laparoscopic cryosurgery of the kidney in the porcine model: an acute histological study. Urology 51:161–166

22. Rukstalis DB, Khorsandi M, Garcia FU, Hoenig DM, Cohen JK (2001) Clinical experience with open renal cryoablation. Urology 57:34–39

Prostate Cryoablation

Bryan J. Donnelly[1] and John C. Rewcastle[2]

Summary. The incidence of prostate cancer in Japan has risen dramatically in the past four decades. This increase, along with the advent of prostate-specific antigen (PSA) screening, has meant that an increasing number of patients are diagnosed at an early stage of the disease, when cure is possible. Currently, radical surgery and external-beam radiation are considered the standards of care for curative treatment of localized disease. Although many patients are helped by these treatment approaches, both are associated with potentially serious complications. Cryoablation is another option in the treatment of localized prostate cancer. The current technique utilizes real-time transrectal ultrasound (TRUS) for guidance and monitoring, multiple cryoprobes, a urethral warming device, multiple thermocouples, and two freeze-thaw cycles. Seven-year outcomes are now available for cryosurgical treatment of primary disease, and they indicate an efficacy similar to that of radical surgery and external-beam radiation in low-risk patients, and possibly superior efficacy in medium- and high-risk patients. Patients who experience a local recurrence following cryoablation can be successfully retreated. Bowel and bladder complications are minimal, and many patients regain the ability to have intercourse. Quality of life has been shown to return to baseline levels within 1 year following the procedure. Cryoablation has been successfully used as salvage therapy in patients with local recurrence, and preliminary evidence suggests that cryoablation may be effective in the treatment of focal disease, where less than the entire gland is targeted.

Keywords. Cryoablation, Cryosurgery, Cryotherapy, Prostate cancer, Review, Prostate carcinoma

[1] Departments of Surgery, Oncology and Urology, Tom Baker Cancer Center, University of Calgary, Alberta, Canada
[2] Department of Radiology, University of Calgary, No. 212, 1011 Glenmore Trail S.W., Calgary, Alberta T2V 4R6, Canada

129

Introduction

Although prostate cancer remains a relatively uncommon cause of cancer death in Japan, the incidence has risen from 0.5 per 100,000 in 1950 to 8.4 per 100,000 in 2001 [1], representing a 17-fold increase in the age-adjusted incidence of the disease. The rising incidence in Japan is a reflection of an increasing worldwide trend. In North America, prostate cancer is the most common cancer in men, and the second most common cause of cancer death [2]. Similarly, a high incidence is seen in many Western countries, which many authors attribute, in part, to diet. As a result of the introduction of prostate-specific antigen (PSA) screening for prostate cancer in the past decade, many more men are now diagnosed with localized disease, when local treatment and cure are possible. At this time, the optimal treatment for localized disease is unclear. There is even debate as to whether or not treatment is advisable. Radical prostatectomy and external-beam radiotherapy are considered the standards of care in the management of localized disease. Brachytherapy and cryoablation are two other forms of local treatment available to this patient population. The current practice in Canada, when advising a patient with localized prostate cancer, is to outline the various treatment options. No treatment is completely effective, and all treatments are associated with a potential negative impact on the patient's quality of life (QOL). Disease characteristics such as the Gleason score, clinical stage, PSA level, number of positive biopsies, and gland size all impact treatment choice. Patient factors such as age, potential life expectancy, sexual activity, and comorbidity also influence treatment selection. In the absence of prospective, randomized clinical trials comparing the efficacy of different therapies for localized prostate cancer, comparative information is based on across-studies comparisons.

The general acceptance of PSA as a surrogate marker of long-term outcome helps in comparing efficacy rates in the literature and guiding treatment selection.

History of Modern Cryoablation

The application of extreme cold for the destruction of superficial lesions has been in use since the mid-1800s. A detailed history of these developments has been documented by Gage [3] and Rubinsky [4]. A cryosurgical milestone occurred in 1961 when Irving Cooper and Arnold Lee [5] successfully built an advanced liquid-nitrogen cryogenic probe. This small-caliber, vacuum-insulated, multilumen probe, which very closely resembles modern liquid cryogen probes, allowed for the initiation of effective, controlled deep-tissue freezing. Gonder et al. [6] were among the first to perform prostatic cryoablation for both benign and malignant disease that caused bladder neck obstruction. They used a single blunt transurethral cryoprobe and monitored their freezing process by digital palpation from the rectum. The technique evolved into a combination of transurethral freezing and an open perineal approach that exposed the apex of the prostate. This approach allowed for separation of the anterior rectal wall from the prostate, thereby significantly reducing the risk of rectal injury [7]. Although the rectum was protected, this approach resulted in significant urinary dysfunction and the development of urethrocutaneous urinary fistulas. However, it did provide sufficient cancer control to prompt further development. A transperineal percutaneous approach was reported in 1974 by Megalli et al. [8]. These authors used a single 6.3-mm sharp-tipped liquid-nitrogen cryoprobe. This cryoprobe was introduced through a small skin incision in the perineum and was guided into the prostate by digital palpation. Freezing, however, continued to be monitored primarily by digital transrectal palpation. Despite the ability of cryoablation to effectively ablate tumor tissue, surgeons remained unable to accurately place the cryoprobes and control the extent of freezing [9]. This resulted in abandonment of the procedure until the advent of real-time ultrasound imaging and guidance. In 1993, Onik et al. [10] reported a significant advancement in prostate cryoablation that utilized three major innovations: the use of real-time transrectal ultrasound (TRUS) monitoring, simultaneous use of multiple ($n = 5$) cryoprobes, and a urethral warming catheter. Current prostate cryosurgical techniques followed directly from these innovations. The current practice of prostate cryoablation employs multiple cryoprobes (6 to 18) that are placed in the prostate transperineally percutaneously, using transrectal ultrasound imaging for guidance and monitoring. Temperature monitoring is carried out by multiple thermocouples placed in and around the prostate, since ultrasound imaging cannot monitor adequate tissue freezing [11].

Technique

The technique used at our institution is a modification of the one originally described by Onik and colleagues [10] and incorporates the advances reported from our center [11, 12]. In our initial experience, patients were treated by a team consisting of a urologist and a radiologist. Currently, most treatments are carried out by a urologist proficient in the use of ultrasound equipment. Prostate cryoablation is usually an in-patient procedure requiring an overnight stay in the hospital, but it may be carried out as an out-patient procedure with same-day discharge. Intravenous antibiotics (cefazolin, gentamicin, and metronidazole) are administered 1 hour preoperatively. The rectum is emptied by repeated use of a fleet enema. The vast majority of patients are treated under spinal anesthetic. The patient is placed in the lithotomy position, and sequential compression devices are applied to the legs preoperatively. Patient positioning is important for providing good access to the perineum, especially if one is using a brachytherapy arm and a computer treatment-planning system. A low lithotomy position is used. The patient's perineum is placed level with the end of the operating table to allow unimpeded access. If the pubic arch is low, an exaggerated lithotomy position can be used to improve transperineal access to the prostate gland. The entire perineum and suprapubic area is prepped with provadone iodine solution, and the patient is draped as for an endoscopic procedure.

A flexible cystoscope is used to visualize the prostate and bladder, to fill the bladder, and to guide the placement of the suprapubic 10 French pigtail catheter. We prefer a suprapubic to a urethral catheter, because we feel that this is easier for the patient, and it avoids irritation of the urethra and prostate during the recovery period. The catheter is removed once the patient's postvoiding residual urine is consistently below 100 ml, typically around 2 weeks postsurgery. Next, a guidewire is inserted into the bladder through the cystoscope, and the cystoscope is removed. A well-lubricated urethral warming catheter (Endocare, Irvine, CA, USA) is introduced through the urethra over the guidewire. The guidewire is removed, and the urethral warming catheter is left in the patient throughout the treatment and for 30 min afterward. Water at 39.5°C is circulated through the warming catheter using a warmer pump system, circulating at a rate of 400 to 500 ml per minute. We routinely add methylene blue dye to this circulating water to aid in rapid identification of any leaks. Some operators initially insert a Foley catheter, replacing it with the warming catheter once the cryoprobes are in place, thereby reducing the risk of puncturing the warming catheter during cryoprobe insertion. A biplane TRUS probe (Aloka, Tokyo, Japan) is inserted into the rectum to visualize and measure the prostate. Intermittent instillation of water into the rectum facilitates good visualization of the prostate. This also distends the rectum to eliminate wrinkles in the anterior rectal wall, which can falsely exaggerate the thickness of the rectal wall.

Six cryoprobes are routinely used, although the number can vary if the prostate is very large, small, or unusually shaped. We refer to the probes by a standard numbering system, which we use in every case (Fig. 1). This system is used because probes are operated sequentially from anterior to posterior, i.e., probes 1 and 2 are operated first, followed by 3 and 4, and then 5 and 6, working from anterior to posterior. This sequencing is utilized to maximize the TRUS visualization during the procedure. If the operator is using 3-mm cryoprobes, probe placement is greatly facilitated by using a rapid access needle/dilator/sheath (Fasttrac, Endocare). This method replaces the original Seldinger technique and significantly reduces the operating time. When the smaller sharp cryoprobes (2.4, 1.8, and 1 mm) are used, they are introduced percutaneously directly into the gland under TRUS visualization. The two anterior sheaths (1 and 2) are initially placed as demonstrated in Fig. 1. The cryoprobes must be less than 10 mm from the edge of the gland to ensure adequate freezing of the periphery. The temperature between the probes will fall more rapidly than the temperature at the edge of the iceball. Anterior cryoprobes can be placed up to 3 cm apart if necessary, whereas all other cryoprobes should be separated by no more than 2 cm (Fig. 1). Sagittal TRUS scanning is used to confirm spatial separation of the cryoprobes, and coronal plane scanning is used to ensure proper positioning of the cryoprobe tip at the base of the prostate. Once in place, the probes are "stuck" while the remaining probes are inserted. "Sticking" refers to lowering the temperature of the probes to −10°C, which results in the cryo-

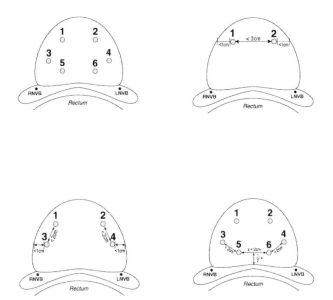

FIG. 1. Cryoprobe placement template. *RNVB*, right neurovascular bundle; *LVNB*, left neurovascular bundle

probe's becoming frozen in place without growing a large iceball. The postero-lateral probes (3 and 4) are placed next. Since the prostate resembles an inverted cone, the probes can be directed laterally from the apex to the base while being inserted, to match the shape of the gland. These must be less than 10 mm from the periphery of the gland. There should be no more than 20 mm between probes 1 and 3 and between probes 2 and 4 to ensure adequate freezing between the probes (Fig. 1). The posteromedial probes (5 and 6) are placed last. Because this placement approaches the warmer, we typically use the coronal plane on the ultrasound probe to place these probes, with the transverse view to fine-tune positioning and ensure adequate separation between cryoprobes. These probes can also be directed laterally when moving from the apex of the gland towards the base, to conform to the shape of the prostate. The iceball generated on these probes is closest to the rectum, and its growth will often dictate the end of the freeze. It is important, therefore, that these probes be placed far enough away from the rectal wall. When the cryoprobes are oriented in the coronal plane, they are placed no more than 2 cm apart, closer to the midline than to the posterior margin of the gland. This ensures good freezing across the midline before the iceball reaches the rectal wall.

In placing the probes, lateral placement is very important, because the tem-perature between the probes is much lower than the temperature at the edge of the iceball. We are always mindful of achieving sufficiently cold temperatures around the gland margin, especially adjacent to the neurovascular bundles where the blood flow is most concentrated.

Thermocouples are a critical part of the cryosurgical procedure, because ultra-sound alone is unreliable in ensuring adequate freezing. A minimum of three and as many as five thermocouples can be placed around the gland: one in each neurovascular bundle (Fig. 1), and one at the gland apex in the midline, just ante-rior to the rectal wall. This is an area that is prone to inadequate freezing and is well documented as an area of high risk for a positive margin. Other thermo-couples can be placed anterior to the gland or at any point where specific tem-peratures need to be achieved. Many cryosurgeons also place a thermocouple in the external sphincter to monitor the temperature in this area. Before initiating the freeze, 30 to 50 ml of sterile saline is injected into the space between the ante-rior rectal wall and the posterior surface of the prostate to separate the two struc-tures. This is a very important step, which greatly facilitates an aggressive freeze in the posterior gland without endangering the rectum. The saline causes good separation and also appears to induce hyperthermia and edema (Fig. 2), even though some of the saline is dispersed during treatment. This practice facilitates a more prolonged freeze posteriorly and at a slower rate, thereby "sculpting" the iceball to the shape of the anterior rectal wall. The freeze is initiated with the two anterior probes. The posterolateral cryoprobes (3 and 4) are turned on when the initial iceball reaches these probes and the iceballs begin to coalesce ante-rior to the urethra. The anterior probes are operated for at least 2 min before probes 3 and 4 are turned on. It is best to begin the freeze slowly, using 50% of the maximum setting for this initial 2-minute period. The rate of freezing is then increased to 75% or 100%. The posteromedial probes (5 and 6) are turned on last. We initially run these probes at 25% and modify the posterolateral probes

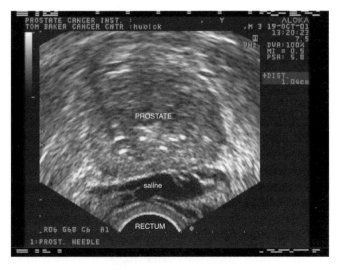

Fig. 2. Ultrasound image of saline injected into the Denonvilliers fascia to increase the separation between the prostate and the posterior rectal wall

(3 and 4) at the same time. The temperature of probes 3 and 4 determines the speed of iceball development on probes 5 and 6. This is the critical part of the procedure, and it is better to proceed slowly, allowing the iceball to grow slowly and therefore conform to the shape of the gland and the anterior rectal wall. The operator should anticipate that when ice bridges across the posterior prostate between the urethra and the rectum, the temperature and behavior of this ice directly anterior to the mid-rectum are influenced by cryoprobes 3 and 4 as well as probes 5 and 6.

At all times, but especially during this part of the procedure, the iceball must be monitored closely to ensure adequate freezing and to protect the anterior rectal wall. The thermocouples are very important, because they relay temperature information much more accurately than the appearance of the iceball. As the iceball approaches the rectal wall, intermittent digital rectal examination (DRE) is a very useful adjunct to TRUS, allowing the surgeon to palpate the anterior rectal wall. It is important to ensure that the mucosa feels soft over the hard iceball lying underneath. On many occasions, TRUS has misled us into believing that there was a very large margin of safety, when DRE revealed the rectum to be very thin but redundantly folded on itself. There will be occasions when the iceball will extend posteriorly to the rectum before the apical thermocouple reaches at least −20°C. In these cases, the edematous reaction to the first freeze will facilitate a more aggressive freeze on the second cycle. Finally, it has been our experience that the operator should continue the freeze longer than he or she might think necessary in order to achieve a truly adequate freeze. As long as the rectum is safe, the operator should strive to achieve an iceball that becomes distinctly flat or even concave to palpation on DRE as it begins to extend laterally around the rectum. Once the first cycle is complete, the argon (the freezing agent) is turned off until the entire prostate is thawed and no ice is visible on ultrasound. Helium (thawing agent) is circulated through the probes to accelerate thawing. This can take between 10 and 30 min, depending on blood flow to the prostate. Before starting the second freeze, it is important to check that none of the cryoprobes have slipped or require repositioning. The second freeze is executed in the same manner as the first. The second freeze consistently progresses faster than the first because of diminished thermal capacity in the previously frozen tissue.

As described above, there are three fundamental steps involved in performing prostate cryoablation. First, a cryoprobe and thermocouple placement strategy is determined. Second, the cryoprobes and thermocouples are placed in the prostate. Finally, the prostate is frozen twice with an interposing complete thaw. Commercially available treatment-planning software, as well as freezing algorithms that control cryoprobe operation based on thermocouple feedback, are now available and greatly facilitate the procedure by aiding in each of these three steps.

Optimization of probe placement is accomplished by capturing an ultrasound image of the prostate. The planning software uses the geometry of the prostate, urethra, and rectal wall to calculate the optimal positions of the cryoprobes and thermocouples. Probes are then inserted through a brachytherapy-like template placed at the perineum. Once this is done, the cryomachine is started in an auto-freeze mode. With the use of real-time temperature feedback from the thermo-couples, the freezing protocol, as described above, is performed, and the flow of argon and helium through the cryoprobes is controlled by the computer.

On completion of the procedure, the cryoprobes are thawed and withdrawn. The urethral warming catheter is left in place for 30 min after the procedure to protect the urethral mucosa against latent freezing and is then withdrawn in the recovery room. Patients at our institution are admitted overnight and discharged the following morning. Many centers perform cryoablation as an outpatient procedure.

Cryoablation as a Primary Treatment for Localized Prostate Cancer

Prostate cancer presents a spectrum of disease ranging from relatively non-aggressive, low-risk disease to very aggressive, high-risk disease. Therefore, assessment of treatment outcome is best done by stratifying patients into those with low-, intermediate-, and high–risk disease, as done by d'Amico et al. [13]. Low risk is defined as T1-2a, Gleason score of 6 or less, and PSA less than 10 ng/ml. Intermediate risk is defined as one of the following: stage higher than T2a, Gleason score greater than 6, or PSA greater than 10 ng/ml. High risk is defined as two or more of the following: stage higher than T2a, Gleason score greater than 6, and PSA greater than 10 ng/ml. Figure 3 (reprinted with permission from Katz and Rewcastle [44]) shows a range of outcomes for the three risk groups from published papers with a minimum 5-year follow-up. These results show excellent outcomes, particularly for patients with higher-risk disease, which is notoriously difficult to treat successfully. Figures 4 and 5, also from Katz and Rewcastle [44], show cryosurgical outcomes compared with those of radical prostatectomy, brachytherapy, and external-beam radiation. Of particular inter-est are the results of cryoablation in intermediate- and high-risk patients. Although the number of publications on cryoablation with 5-year follow-up is limited, and the patient numbers are low in comparison to those undergoing surgery and external-beam radiation, the published results are at least equiva-lent, if not superior, to those for all forms of radiotherapy and surgery in moderate- and high-risk patients.

Posttreatment biopsies have been performed by many authors reporting the results of cryoablation as primary treatment for localized prostate cancer (Table 1). Bahn et al. [14] report an overall positive biopsy rate of 13% in patients, with a mean follow-up of 5.72 years. Our own series shows that 72 of 73 patients exhib-ited negative biopsies. This negative biopsy rate was achieved, in part, as the result of repeat cryoablation in 11 patients. The ability to retreat the patient is one of the advantages of cryoablation. In our own pilot series of 76 patients,

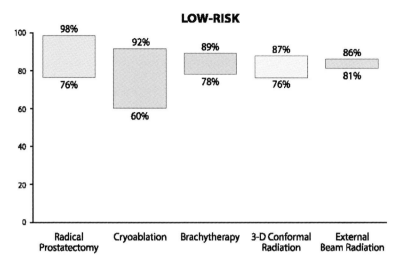

FIG. 3. Comparison of biochemical disease-free rates as reported in the literature since 1992 for low-risk disease

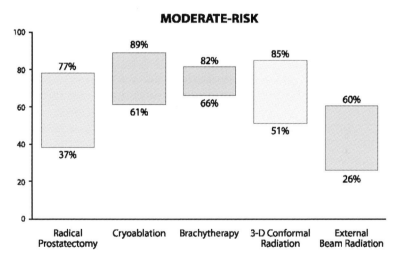

FIG. 4. Comparison of biochemical disease-free rates as reported in the literature since 1992 for moderate-risk disease

follow-up biopsy was initially positive in 11 cases. Four of these 11 were from the first 10 patients we ever treated, and these 10 patients had a single freeze cycle. The remaining 7 positive biopsies were found in the subsequent 66 patients. Patients with positive biopsies were retreated, and eventually 72 of the 73 patients from this series who underwent biopsy were biopsy negative. Reported biopsy outcomes for brachytherapy, conformal-beam radiotherapy, and external-

TABLE 1. Positive biopsy results observed following radiation therapy and cryoablation

Study	Therapy	N	Pretreatment PSA (ng/ml)	Gleason score	Clinical T stage	Median follow-up	% positive biopsy
Stock et al. 1996 [17]	Brachytherapy	97	75% < 20	82% < 7	T1–T2	18mo	26%
Ragde et al. 1997 [15]	Brachytherapy	126	78.7% < 10; median 5.0	2–6	T1–T2	7yr	5%[a]
Ragde et al. 1998 [16]	Brachytherapy	152	Median 11.0	91% < 8	98% < T3	10yr	15%
Zelefsky et al. 1998 [51]	3D-CRT	743	Median 15	81< 8	T1–T3	>30mo	48%
Dinges et al. 1998 [19]	XRT	82	Median 14.0		T2–T3	24mo	27%
Crook et al. 1998 [18]	XRT	102			T1–T3	40mo	20%[b]
Babaian et al. 1995 [24]	XRT	31	70% > 10		T1–T3	51mo	71%
Laverdiere et al. 1997 [22]	XRT	120	Median 11.2	24.3% > 6	T1–T3	24mo	62%
Ljung et al. 1995 [23]	XRT	55		35% > 6	T1–T3	6.8yr	67%
Bahn et al. 2002 [14]	Cryoablation	590	24.5% > 10	58.4% > 6	T1–T4	5.72yr	13%
Donnelly et al. 2002 [24]	Cryoablation	76	38% > 10	56% > 6	T1–T3	5.1yr	15%

PSA, prostate-specific antigen; 3D-CRT, three-dimensional conformal radiation therapy; TCAP, targeted cryoablation of the prostate; XRT, external-beam radiation therapy

[a] 13% indeterminate
[b] 15% indeterminate

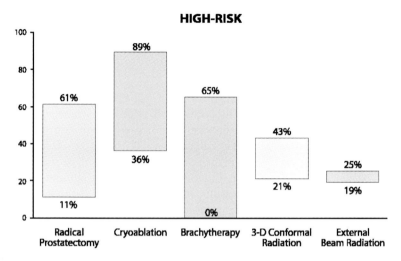

Fig. 5. Comparison of biochemical disease-free rates as reported in the literature since 1992 for high-risk disease

beam radiotherapy yield significantly lower results. The rate of positive biopsies following brachytherapy [15–17] ranges from 5% to 26%, with follow-up periods ranging from 18 months to 10 years. The series reporting the 5% positive biopsy rate was composed solely of patients in the low-risk category [15]. Crook and Bunting [18] reported a 48% positive biopsy rate in their series of conformal-beam radiotherapy in patients with more than 30 months of follow-up, and other series report rates of positive biopsy between 20% and 71%, with follow-up periods ranging from 2 to 6.8 years [19–23].

Morbidity

With any cancer therapy, there is a fine balance between aggressive disease eradication and increased treatment-induced morbidity, with a corresponding negative impact on QOL. This balance applies to any of the treatment modalities available for localized prostate cancer. As the technique of prostate cryoablation is evolving, and as experience with this modality is increasing, the morbidity reported has steadily declined. Sexual dysfunction and bladder and bowel changes have the greatest negative impact on the lives of prostate cancer patients following treatment for their disease. Historically, urorectal fistula formation was a major concern with prostate cryoablation. Advances in technology and technique have virtually eliminated this concern with cryoablation. Among four recent publications [14, 24–26], only one found rectal complications [14], with a fistula rate of less than 0.1%. Incontinence in these series ranged from 1.3% to 5.4%, and postoperative impotence ranged from 82.4% to 100% in previously potent men. In our own series at 3-year follow-up, 47% of men sexually active prior to treatment had resumed sexual intercourse.

Quality of Life

QOL outcome is increasingly being recognized as an important component in evaluating treatment for prostate cancer. In patients for whom different treatments are deemed to be similarly effective, QOL outcomes frequently will determine the choice of treatment from the patient's point of view. We have recently published the long-term outcomes of QOL assessment in patients treated with cryoablation. The results indicate that the outcomes are comparable or superior to QOL outcome following other treatments [27, 28]. Two validated and commonly used measuring instruments were used to follow the patients: the Colon Functional Assessment of Prostate Cancer (FACT-P) and the Sexuality Follow-up Questionnaire (SFQ). At 1 year following treatment, patient QOL measurements had returned to pretreatment levels in all areas, with the exception of sexual functioning. At 3 years posttreatment, baseline levels remained constant, with no delayed-onset morbidity. The major change observed at 3 years was the significant improvement in sexual functioning, with 47% of men who were potent before treatment recovering the ability to achieve intercourse. The use of QOL assessments has been greatly enhanced by the work of Litwin et al. [29], who measured 5-year outcomes following radical surgery, radiotherapy, and observation. Similar measurements have been carried out by Krupski et al. [30], who performed QOL measurements 9 months following treatment in brachytherapy patients. The QOL outcomes from our own series compare favorably with both of these published reports (Table 2). Of note is the absence of delayed-onset morbidity following cryoablation.

Long-Term Outcome

Long-term follow-up is essential to fully judge the efficacy of treatment for localized prostate cancer. Ten to 15 years of follow-up data is considered optimal, and follow-up information of this duration is available in a small number of series for both radical surgery and external-beam radiation. At this time, 7-year results are the longest available in the literature for cryoablation [14]. Until 10-year results are available, the case for long-term efficacy of cryoablation cannot be conclusively made. Nonetheless, the 7-year results have demonstrated a durable efficacy equivalent to that of other therapies for low-risk disease. In the treatment of intermediate- and high-risk disease, cryoablation may actually confer a superior benefit compared with other treatment modalities. What can explain this favorable comparison? The higher the Gleason score, the greater the likelihood of a positive margin at the time of radical prostatectomy [31]. Similarly, a higher Gleason score is associated with less effective radiation therapy outcome

TABLE 2. Quality of life of men treated with cryoablation compared with men undergoing radical prostatectomy, radiation, brachytherapy, or observation[a]

Variable	Cryoablation (N = 64)[b]	Surgery (N = 98)[b]	Radiation (N = 60)[b]	Brachytherapy (N = 41)[c]	Observation (N = 60)[b]
FACT-P scales	Mean	Mean	Mean	Mean	Mean
Physical well-being	26.1	25.4	24.9	25.4	25.2
Social/family well-being	21.9	21.6	21.6	14.9	21.1
Emotional well-being	18.1	16.6	17.3	21.3	16.6
Functional well-being	24.6	20.9	21.2	23.6	20.7
Relationship with doctor	7.5	6.5	6.5	NA[d]	6.3

[a] Higher scores indicate better QOL outcomes at 3 years
[b] Litwin et al. [29], average follow-up, 5 years
[c] Krupski et al. [30], 9 months follow-up
[d] NA, not available

[32, 33]. With cryoablation, the freezing process is always extended beyond the surgical margin of the gland, thereby overcoming this limitation of radical surgery. Unlike radiotherapy, which destroys the target tissue by damaging the cell nucleus, cryoablation destroys the target tissue by the physical disruption induced by the formation of intracellular ice. It is for this reason that tumor grade is not an important factor affecting the ability of cryoablation to destroy the cells. The only limitation on the use of cryoablation in higher-grade cases is whether the malignant cells are confined to the prostate and the immediate local area or have metastasized.

Salvage Cryoablation

The treatment of locally recurrent prostate cancer following radiation therapy (either external-beam radiotherapy or brachytherapy) with cryoablation is frequently referred to as salvage cryoablation. Radiation therapy, in the form of either external-beam radiotherapy or brachytherapy, is used to treat large numbers of men with localized prostate cancer in North America each year. Unfortunately, 25% to 93% of these patients have a relapse of their disease, many with isolated local recurrences [34, 35]. The treatment options are limited: salvage radical prostatectomy carries a high risk of significant complications, and hormonal therapy is palliative and not curative [36–38]. Over the past 10 years, cryoablation has been increasingly used in this group of patients. Although early reports were discouraging due to the high rate of significant complications [39–41], more recent reports validate the benefit of this treatment, with significantly less morbidity than that originally reported [42, 43]. These improved results can be attributed to increased experience and technological advances in this setting. Universal use of an effective urethral warming catheter in all centers has led to substantial reductions in morbidity. The use of these devices was initially restricted by the Food and Drug Administration (FDA), which led to a high incidence of complications.

Patient Selection

It has become apparent over the past 10 years that careful patient selection is vitally important to ensure optimal outcomes. Initially, patients with bulky, localized recurrent cancers and those with significantly elevated PSA levels were treated with the hope of salvaging their condition. As pointed out by Katz and Rewcastle [44] and by Chin et al. [43], selection criteria that increase the likelihood that the recurrence will be confined to the prostate are of paramount importance. Therefore, patients with PSA levels less than 10ng/ml and with PSA doubling times greater than 1 year are those best suited for this procedure. Similarly, patients with nonbulky disease are more likely to be treated successfully. Higher Gleason scores prior to radiation or at the time of recurrence indicate a greater likelihood of distant disease and subsequent failure of this localized treatment. Patients who have had a prior transurethral resection of the prostate (TURP) should be advised of the 75% to 80% risk of developing posttreatment incontinence. None of these factors should absolutely exclude a patient from salvage cryoablation, but they allow the surgeon to advise the patient appropriately regarding the potential risks and benefits of the treatment.

Technique

The technique in salvage treatment is similar to that in primary treatment. Generally speaking, the prostate gland is somewhat smaller and the blood flow to the gland is not as good as in the primary cases. As a result of this, the freezing process tends to proceed more rapidly, and the operator must bear this in mind. Also, because the anterior rectal wall has frequently been adversely affected by the radiation therapy, particular care has to be taken to ensure that the anterior rectal wall is not frozen during treatment. There is definitely a higher risk of developing urethrorectal fistulas after salvage cryoablation than after primary cryoablation [39, 45, 46]. In some patients, it may not be possible to bring the thermocouples to −40°C before the iceball begins to invade the anterior rectal wall. In these case, the preservation of the anterior rectal wall must be the primary consideration. The use of a thermocouple placed in the external sphincter has been shown to significantly reduce the incidence of postoperative incontinence, because this aids the operator in preventing the temperature at the external sphincter from going below +15°C [42].

TABLE 3. Results of salvage cryoablation studies reported in the literature

Author	N	Incontinence	Rectal injury	BRFS
Miller et al. [46]	33	9%	0%	40%
Pisters et al. [39]	150	73%	NA	31%
Lee et al. [52]	46	9%	8.7%	53%
Cespedes et al. [53]	107	28%	NA	NA
Chin et al. [54]	118	6.7%	3.3%	35%
Ghafar et al. [42]	38	7.9%	0%	74%
Saliken et al. [55]	31	6%	0%	80%[a]

BRFS, biochemical recurrence-free survival; NA, not available

[a] $61\% \leq 0.3\,\mathrm{ng/ml}$, $80\% \leq 1.0\,\mathrm{ng/ml}$

Results

As with all therapies for prostate cancer, PSA is used as a surrogate for treatment success or failure. Different authors report different PSA thresholds and cutoffs, ranging from less than 0.3 to less than 1.0 ng/ml. Table 3 shows the results of salvage cryoablation studies reported in the literature. These results incorporate early experience with this modality and include many patients with either very elevated PSA levels or bulky disease prior to the cryosurgical procedure. With increasing experience and better selection criteria, the results can be expected to further improve. The incidence of incontinence and rectal injury reported in earlier series has been significantly reduced. Nonetheless, it is to be expected that the incidence of complications following salvage cryoablation will be higher than the complication rate for primary treatment.

The Future

Unlike radical prostatectomy and external-beam radiation, cryoablation can be performed in a targeted area of the prostate. Of necessity, the entire gland is removed during radical prostatectomy. Likewise, the entire gland is irradiated during external-beam radiation. Although most prostate cancers are multifocal [47], there is debate about the significance of some of these lesions. Villers et al. [48] reported that 80% of incidental lesions were less than 0.5 ml, suggesting that many of the multifocal tumors, other than the dominant cancer, may not be clinically significant. Rukstalis et al. [49] suggested that significant cancer could be eliminated in 79% of men if the index lesion was targeted. Efforts are under way to help identify men with single lesions, thereby selecting patients who would be candidates for focal cryoablation.

One such study was reported recently by Onik et al. [50]. The side of the prostate with demonstrable cancer was aggressively frozen, and a more conservative freeze was performed on the opposite side. In this way, a reduction in morbidity and preservation of the neurovascular bundle were facilitated. All patients were biopsied, and no patient had residual cancer on biopsy. The mean follow-up time was 36 months. Seven of nine patients (77%) had erections sufficient for intercourse. Further work needs to be done in this area, but it appears to hold promise for the future. If areas of cancer can be visualized by a new imaging modality, this will further enhance this potential advantage of cryoablation.

A variant of the cryosurgical ablation methods described above involves the use of gas-driven (rather than deep-frozen liquid gas) probes that are smaller in diameter. Termed Seednet, 12 to 17 of the 17-gauge (1.47-mm) cryoneedles are placed into the prostate through a brachytherapy-like template. The largest study published to date involved 106 patients with localized prostate cancer [26]. Failure was defined as an inability to reach a PSA nadir of 0.4 ng/ml or less. At 3 months and 12 months postsurgery, 81% and 75% were free from biochemical failure, respectively. Complications included sloughing (5%), incontinence requiring pads (3%), urge incontinence (5%), urinary retention (3.3%), and rectal discomfort (2.6%). Follow-up biopsy was not performed. Although these results are encouraging, caution should be exercised in their interpretation until more mature outcomes are available, as it is possible that the temperatures generated may not be as low as with larger probes.

References

1. National Cancer Center Japan. Cancer Statistics in Japan 2003. Available at: www.ncc.go.jp/en/statistics/2003/data05.pdf. Accessed January 24, 2004. Last update 1/5/04
2. American Cancer Society (ACS). Cancer Facts and Figures 2004. Available at www.cancer.org/docroot/STT/stt_0.asp. Accessed January 24, 2004
3. Gage AA (1998) History of cryosurgery. Semin Surg Oncol 14:99–109
4. Rubinsky B (2000) Cryosurgery. Annu Rev Biomed Eng 2:157–187
5. Cooper IS, Lee AS (1961) Cryostatic congelation: a system for producing a limited, controlled region of cooling or freezing of biologic tissues. J Nerv Ment Dis 133:259–263
6. Gonder MJ, Soanes WA, Shulman S (1966) Cryosurgical treatment of the prostate. Invest Urol 3:372–378
7. Soanes WA, Gonder MJ (1968) Use of cryosurgery in prostatic cancer. J Urol 99:793–797
8. Megalli MR, Gursel EO, Veenema RJ (1974) Closed perineal cryosurgery in prostatic cancer. New probe and technique. Urology 4:220–222
9. Bonney WW, Fallon B, Gerber WL (1982) Cryosurgery in prostatic cancer: survival. Urology 19:37–42
10. Onik GM, Cohen JK, Reyes GD, et al (1993) Transrectal ultrasound-guided percutaneous radical cryosurgical ablation of the prostate. Cancer 72:1291–1299
11. Steed J, Saliken JC, Donnelly BJ, Ali-Ridha NH (1997) Correlation between thermosensor temperature and transrectal ultrasonography during prostate cryoablation. Can Assoc Radiol J 48:186–190
12. Saliken JC, Donnelly BJ, Ernst S, Rewcastle J, Wiseman D (2001) Prostate cryotherapy: practicalities and applications from the Calgary experience. Can Assoc Radiol J 52:165–173

13. D'Amico AV, Whittington R, Malkowicz SB, et al (1998) Biochemical outcome after radical prostatectomy, external beam radiation therapy, or interstitial radiation therapy for clinically localized prostate cancer. JAMA 16:969–974

14. Bahn DK, Lee F, Badalament R, Kumar A, Greski J, Chernick M (2002) Targeted cryoablation of the prostate: 7-year outcomes in the primary treatment of prostate cancer. Urology 60(Suppl 2A):3–11

15. Ragde H, Blasko JC, Grimm PD, et al (1997) Interstitial iodine-125 radiation without adjuvant therapy in the treatment of clinically localized prostate carcinoma. Cancer 80:442–453

16. Ragde H, Elgamal A-A, Snow PB, et al (1998) Ten-year disease free survival after transperineal sonography-guided iodine-125 brachytherapy with or without 45-gray external beam irradiation in the treatment of patients with clinically localized, low to high Gleason grade prostate carcinoma. Cancer 83:989–1001

17. Stock RG, Stone NN, DeWyngaert JK, et al (1996) Prostate specific antigen findings and biopsy results following interactive ultrasound guided transperineal brachytherapy for early stage prostate carcinoma. Cancer 77:2386–2392

18. Crook JM, Bunting PS (1998) Percent free prostate-specific antigen after radiotherapy for prostate cancer. Urology 52:100–105

19. Dinges S, Deger S, Koswig S, et al (1998) High-dose rate interstitial with external beam irradiation for localized prostate cancer: results of a prospective trial. Radiother Oncol 48:197–202

20. Crook JM, Bunting PS (1998) Percent free prostate-specific antigen after radiotherapy for prostate cancer. Urology 52:100–105

21. Babaiain RJ, Kojima M, Saitoh M, et al (1995) Detection of residual prostate cancer after external radiotherapy. Cancer 75:2153–2158

22. Laverdiere J, Gomez JL, Cusan L, et al (1997) Beneficial effect of combining hormonal therapy administered prior and following external beam radiation therapy for localized prostate cancer. Int J Radiat Oncol Biol Phys 37:247–252

23. Ljung G, Norberg M, Hansson H, et al (1995) Transrectal ultrasonically-guided core biopsies in the assessment of local cure of prostatic cancer after radical external beam radiotherapy. Acta Oncologica 34:945–952

24. Donnelly BJ, Saliken JC, Ernst DS, Ali-Ridha N, Brasher PMA, Robinson JW, Rewcastle JC (2002) A prospective trial of cryosurgical ablation of the prostate: five-year results. Urology 60:645–649

25. Ellis DS (2002) Cryosurgery as primary treatment for localized prostate cancer. A community hospital experience 60(Suppl 2A):34–39

26. Han KR, Cohen JK, Miller RJ, et al (2003) Treatment of organ confined prostate cancer with third generation cryosurgery: preliminary multicenter experience. J Urol 170(4 Pt 1):1126–1130

27. Robinson JW, Donnelly BJ, Saliken JC, Weber BA, Ernst S, Rewcastle JC (2002) Quality of life and sexuality of men with prostate cancer 3 years after cryosurgery. Urology 60(Suppl 2A):12–18

28. Robinson JW, Saliken JC, Donnelly BJ, Barnes P, Guyn L (1999) Quality-of-life outcomes for men treated with cryosurgery for localized prostate carcinoma. Cancer 86:1793–1801.

29. Litwin MS, Hays RD, Fink A, et al (1995) Quality-of-life outcomes in men treated for localized prostate cancer. JAMA 273:129–135

30. Krupski T, Petroni GR, Bissonette EA, et al (2000) Quality-of-life comparison of radical prostatectomy and interstitial brachytherapy in the treatment of clinically localized prostate cancer. Urology 55:736–742
31. El-Feel A, Davis JW, Deger S, et al (2003) Positive margins after laparoscopic radical prostatectomy: a prospective study of 100 cases performed by 4 different surgeons. Eur Urol 43:622–626
32. Kuban DA, Thames HD, Levy LB, et al (2003) Long-term multi-institutional analysis of stage T1-T2 prostate cancer treated with radiotherapy in the PSA era. Int J Radiat Oncol Biol Phys 57:915–928
33. Martinez A, Gonzalez J, Spencer W, et al (2003) Conformal high dose rate brachytherapy improves biochemical control and cause-specific survival in patients with prostate cancer and poor prognostic factors. J Urol 2003:974–979; discussion 979–980
34. de la Taille A, Hayek O, Benson M, et al (2000) Salvage cryotherapy for recurrent prostate cancer after radiation therapy: the Colombia experience. Urology 55:79–84
35. Prestige BR, Kaplan I, Cox RS, Bagshaw MA (1994) Predictors of survival after a positive post-irradiation prostate biopsy. Int J Radiat Oncol Biol Phys 28:17–22
36. Rogers E, Ohori M, Kassabian VS, et al (1995) Salvage radical prostatectomy: outcome measured by serum prostate specific antigen levels. J Urol 153:104–110
37. Lerner SE, Blute ML, Zincke H (1995) Critical evaluation of salvage surgery for radiorecurrent/resistant prostate cancer. J Urol 154:1103–1109
38. Corral DA, Pisters LL, von Eschenbach AC (1996) Treatment options for localized recurrence of prostate cancer following radiation therapy. Urol Clin N Am 23:677–684
39. Pisters LL, von Eschenbach AC, Scott SM, et al (1997) The efficacy and complications of salvage cryotherapy of the prostate. J Urol 157:921–925
40. Chodak GW (1993) Cryosurgery of the prostate revisited. Cancer 72:1145–1146
41. Bales GT, Williams MJ, Sinner M, et al (1995) Short-term outcomes after cryosurgical ablation of the prostate in men with recurrent prostate carcinoma following radiation therapy. Urology 46:676–680
42. Ghafar MA, Johnson CW, de la Taille A, et al (2001) Salvage cryotherapy using an argon based system for locally recurrent prostate cancer after radiation therapy: the Columbia experience. J Urol 166:1333–1338
43. Chin JL, Pautler SE, Mouraviev V, et al (2001) Results of salvage cryoablation of the prostate after radiation: identifying predictors of treatment failure and complications. J Urol 165:1937–1942
44. Katz AE, Rewcastle JC (2003) The current and potential role of cryoablation as a primary therapy for localized prostate cancer. Curr Oncol Rep 5:231–238
45. Bales GT, Williams MJ, Sinner M, et al (1995) Short-term outcomes after cryosurgical ablation of the prostate in men with recurrent prostate carcinoma following radiation therapy. Urology 46:676–680
46. Miller RJ, Cohen JK, Shuman B, Merlotti LA (1996) Percutaneous, transperineal cryosurgery of the prostate as salvage therapy for post radiation recurrence of adenocarcinoma. Cancer 77:1510–1514
47. Epstein JI, Walsh PC, Akingba G, et al (1999) The significance of prior benign needle biopsies in men subsequently diagnosed with prostate cancer. J Urol 162:1649–1652
48. Villers A, McNeal JE, Freiha FS, et al (1992) Multiple cancers in the prostate. Morphologic features of clinically recognized vs. incidental tumors. Cancer 70:2312–2318
49. Rukstalis DB, Goldknoph JL, Crowley EM, et al (2002) Prostate cryoablation: a scientific rationale for future modifications. Urology 60(2 Suppl 1):19–25

50. Onik G, Narayan P, Vaughan D, et al (2002) Focal "nerve-sparing" cryosurgery for treatment of primary prostate cancer: a new approach to preserving potency. Urology 60:109–114
51. Zelefsky MJ, Leibel SA, Gaudin PB, et al (1998) Dose escalation with three-dimensional conformal radiation therapy affects the outcome of prostate cancer. Int J Radiat Oncol Biol Phys 41:491–500
52. Lee F, Bahn DK, McHugh TA, et al (1997) Cryosurgery of prostate cancer. Use of adjuvant hormonal therapy and temperature monitoring: a one year follow-up. Anticancer Res 17:1511–1515
53. Cespedes RD, Pisters LL, von Eschenbach AC, McGuire EJ (1997) Long-term follow-up of incontinence and obstruction after salvage cryosurgical ablation of the prostate: results in 143 patients. J Urol 157:237–240
54. Chin JL, Pautler SE, Mouraviev V, et al (2001) Results of salvage cryoablation of the prostate after radiation: identifying predictors of treatment failure and complications. J Urol 165:1937–1942
55. Saliken JC, Donnelly BJ, Ernst DS, et al (in press) Efficacy and complications of salvage cryosurgery for recurrent prostate carcinoma after radiotherapy

Tumor Control Outcome and Tolerance of Permanent Interstitial Implantation for Patients with Clinically Localized Prostate Cancer

Michael J. Zelefsky

Summary. There have been significant improvements in the way prostate brachytherapy is currently performed, which have directly led to superior biochemical control rates and reduced side effect profiles. Transperineal ultrasound-guided approaches have replaced the open retropubic technique, and the 15-year results now available indicate excellent biochemical outcomes for patients with early-stage, low-risk cancer. In general, PSA relapse-free survival outcomes for favorable-risk disease have been reported to be approximately 90%, which is comparable to outcomes achieved with other interventions such as radical prostatectomy and high-dose conformal external-beam radiotherapy. Although urinary obstructive symptoms are commonly reported as acute effects observed immediately after therapy, these effects gradually resolve with time. Newer strategies in prostate brachytherapy are exploring techniques that will probably further enhance the accuracy of seed implantation with intraoperative planning methods. These approaches provide three-dimensional target and normal tissue reconstruction in the operating room during the procedure, which in turn can improve the accuracy of the seed placement and reduce the radiation dose levels delivered to the urethra and rectum. Reports of the use of these techniques indicate reduced urinary symptoms along with excellent biochemical control rates. Recently, methods have been developed to fuse the coordinates of biologic-based imaging abnormalities such as magnetic resonance spectroscopy on intraoperative ultrasound images and target higher doses to these regions. Real-time seed identification with reintegration of this information into the treatment plan in a dynamic mode will further enhance the precision of this procedure and likely lead to a further improvement in the quality of life among patients treated with prostate brachytherapy.

Keywords. Prostate Cancer, Brachytherapy, Preplanning, Intraoperative Planning, Biochemical Control, Toxicity

Memorial Sloan-Kettering Cancer Center, New York, USA

Introduction

Permanent interstitial implantation has become a standard treatment option for patients with localized prostate cancer. Over the last 30 years, significant improvements in implantation techniques have emerged, which have dramatically improved the outcomes with this treatment intervention. Ultrasound-guided transperineal techniques have replaced the open retropubic implantation approach, and the implantation procedure has become more precise. Ten-year biochemical outcomes for favorable-risk disease compare favorably with the excellent results observed after radical prostatectomy and high-dose conformal external-beam radiotherapy. Recently, intraoperative treatment planning has been introduced, which provides the opportunity for planning the implantation dose delivery in the operating room. These exciting developments have already begun paving the way for enhancing the accuracy of prostate brachytherapy and minimizing the dose delivered to the surrounding normal tissue structures.

This review will highlight the indications and contraindications of permanent seed implantation for patients with localized prostate cancer, and review the published outcomes and expected tolerance profiles for this treatment. In addition, new developments, such as intraoperative planning and the potential for integration of functional imaging information, such as magnetic resonance imaging and spectroscopy, into brachytherapy treatment planning will be discussed.

Brachytherapy Treatment Planning: Standard Techniques and New Developments

The standard technique used for prostate brachytherapy planning is a preplanning method. With this approach, transrectal ultrasound imaging is obtained several days to weeks before the planned procedure to measure the prostate volume. A computerized plan is generated from the transverse ultrasound images, which will in turn demonstrate the optimal location of seeds within the gland to deliver the prescription dose to the prostate. Several days to weeks later, the implantation procedure is performed, and needles are placed through a perineal template according to the coordinates calculated by the preplan. Needle placement is performed under ultrasound guidance, and the radioactive seeds are individually deposited within the needle with the aid of an applicator or with preloaded seeds on a semirigid strand containing the preplanned number of seeds.

Although a preplanning implantation technique has been associated with excellent clinical outcomes, there are some limitations to this approach. These include the technical difficulties associated with matching the exact configurations of the prostate, rectum, and bladder of the preplan obtained in the unanesthetized patient compared with the patient's anatomy during the operative procedure. Consequently, intraoperative adjustments of seed and needle placements are frequently required, and the actual postimplantation dose distribution will not always resemble the idealized preplan. In addition, intraprostatic needle placement causes distortion and edema of the gland, which could lead to significant discrepancies between the preplan anatomic geometry and the actual anatomic conditions during the procedure [1, 2]. At the same time, such deviations may lead to an unintentional increase in the dose delivered to normal tissue structures such as the urethra and rectum, increasing the risks of treatment-related complications.

At Memorial Sloan-Kettering Cancer Center an intraoperative conformal optimization and planning system for ultrasound-based implantation has been used since 1996, which obviates the need for preplanning [3]. This technique involves an inverse-planning conformal optimization system that incorporates acceptable dose ranges allowed within the target volume as well as dose constraints for the rectal wall and urethra. An ultrasound probe is positioned in the rectum, and the prostate and normal anatomy are identified. Needles are inserted through the perineal template and positioned at the periphery of the prostate. The prostate is subsequently scanned from apex to base, and these 0.5-cm images are transferred to the treatment planning system using a PC-based video capture system. On the computer monitor, the prostate contours and the urethra are digitized on each axial image with a 5-mm margin. Needle positions are identified on each image, and their coordinates are incorporated into a genetic algorithm optimization program [4, 5]. After the optimization program has identified the optimal seed-loading pattern and the dose calculations have been completed, isodose displays are superimposed on each transverse ultrasound image and carefully evaluated. Dose-volume histograms for the target volume, rectum, and urethra are also carefully assessed. The entire planning process from the contouring of images to the generation of the seed loading pattern requires approximately 10 minutes. The seeds are then loaded with a standard applicator.

Several comparative analyses have indicated improvements of target coverage with an intraoperative approach compared with a preplanned approach [3, 6, 7]. In a report from our institution [3], the median volume of the prostate target receiving the prescription dose (V100) was 96%. In contrast, the V100 for a computed tomographic (CT) preplan approach was 86% ($p < 0.001$). A multivariate analysis determined that the intraoperative conformal technique (compared with other techniques) was an independent predictor of improved target coverage for each dosimetric parameter analyzed ($p < 0.001$). The maximum and average urethral doses were significantly reduced when this intraoperative technique was introduced (Fig. 1).

Indications and Contraindications for Permanent Prostate Implantation

The ideal candidates for permanent interstitial implantation are those with favorable-risk prognostic features who have a high likelihood of organ-confined

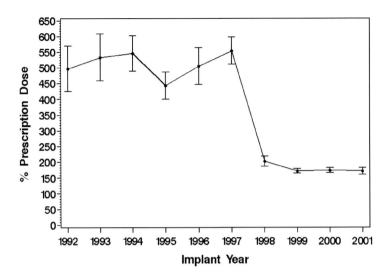

F<small>IG</small>. 1. Maximum urethral dose

disease. This group includes those with prostate-specific antigen (PSA) levels ≤10 ng/ml and with Gleason scores <7. Although not essential for staging, pretreatment magnetic resonance imaging (MRI) of the prostate with endorectal coil may be helpful in the assessment of the integrity of the prostatic capsule as well as the geometry of the gland. Such information may be invaluable in the planning aspects of transperineal implantation (TPI), as well as determining whether a patient is a candidate for the procedure. The prostate gland size should preferably be less than 60 cm³. With larger gland sizes, the pubic arch may interfere with needle placement to the anterolateral portions of the gland, resulting in inadequate coverage of the target volume. In addition, larger glands require more seeds and activity to achieve coverage of the gland with the prescription dose, resulting in a concomitant increase in the central urethral doses and potentially increasing the risk of urinary morbidity. One report indicated that patients with median lobe hyperplasia have a higher incidence of acute urinary symptoms after prostate brachytherapy [8]. The size of the prostate can be effectively reduced with combined androgen blockade therapy. A reduction in volume of approximately 30% is often observed after three months of androgen deprivation.

A prior transurethral resection (TURP) may increase the risks of urinary morbidity after permanent seed implantation [9, 10]. In these patients implantation should be performed with caution. Using a uniform loading seed pattern, Blasko et al. [10] reported an increased incidence of incontinence and superficial urethral necrosis after permanent interstitial implantation among patients with a prior history of TURP. Wallner et al. [11] observed a three-year actuarial incidence of incontinence of 6% among 11 patients who underwent TURP prior to TPI. Stone et al. [12] reported on 43 patients treated with prostate brachytherapy using a modified peripheral seed loading technique. Although these authors observed no cases of urinary incontinence, the four-year incidence of superficial urethral necrosis was 16%. As noted above, patients with preexisting urinary obstructive symptoms are more likely to experience acute urinary morbidity after seed implantation and need to be appropriately counseled regarding this possibility.

Patients with relative contraindications for external-beam radiotherapy may be more suitable for prostate brachytherapy. These include patients with bilateral hip replacements where CT-based treatment planning is technically difficult due to the substantial artifact created by the prostheses, which preclude adequate visualization of the target volume. Ultrasound-based seed implantation would be an appropriate alternative for such patients. In most cases, patients with hip prostheses are able to tolerate the extended dorsal lithotomy position for adequate perineal exposure during the procedure. Patients in whom the small bowel is in close proximity to the prostate volume are not ideal candidates for high-dose three-dimensional conformal radiotherapy (CRT) and are better suited for seed implantation due to the lower doses to the bowel expected with the latter treatment intervention. In addition, brachytherapy appears to be safe for patients with a history of inflammatory bowel disease (IBD), a condition that represents a relative contraindication for external-beam radiotherapy [13].

Biochemical and Disease Control Outcomes with Low Dose Rate (LDR) Brachytherapy

Grimm et al. [14] reported the outcome of 125 patients treated between 1988 and 1990 with TPI using I-125 and followed for a median of 81 months. A PSA relapse in that report was defined as three consecutive PSA elevations above the nadir PSA level. Among patients defined as having low-risk disease (PSA <10 ng/ml, Gleason score <7, and clinical stage ≤T2b) the 10-year PSA relapse-free survival (RSF) outcome was 87%. Improved long-term outcomes were noted for both favorable- and intermediate-risk patients who were treated after the physicians' initial learning curve was achieved compared with the outcome for the initial patients treated at the center [43]. Blasko et al. [15] reported the outcome of 230 patients treated with Pd-103, with a median follow-up of 41 months. Most patients in this report had favorable risk features, whereas only approximately 30% and 20%, respectively, of the patients had Gleason scores >6 and PSA levels >10 ng/ml. The seven-year PSA RFS (with relapse defined as two consecutive rising PSA values) was 83%. Postimplantation biopsies were performed on 201 patients. The incidence of negative, indeterminate, and positive postimplant biopsies was 80%, 17%, and 3%, respectively [16].

Investigators from the Mount Sinai School of Medicine reported eight-year outcomes of I-125 implantation for 243 patients with a minimum follow-up of five years [17]. The eight-year PSA relapse-free survival outcome for patients with low-risk disease (stage T2a or less, Gleason score <7, and PSA <10 ng/ml) was 88%. Among patients with intermediate-risk features (stage T2b, Gleason score 7, or initial PSA levels 10–20 ng/ml) and unfavorable-risk characteristics (two or more adverse features or Gleason score ≥8, or PSA >20 ng/ml), the eight-year biochemical outcomes were 81% and 65%, respectively. In a subset analysis, among patients with low-risk disease who had an optimal dose based on retrospective postimplantation dosimetry evaluation delivered with the implant (D90 > 140 Gy; $n = 49$), the PSA RFS at eight years was 94%, compared with 75% for patients ($n = 23$) who received suboptimal dose levels with the implant ($p = 0.02$).

Using the collected data from several institutions, Kattan et al. [18] designed a nomogram using a Cox proportional-hazards analysis to predict five-year biochemical outcomes after permanent interstitial brachytherapy alone. The nomogram approach for risk prediction takes into account the many variables known to have an impact on the clinical outcome, such as the PSA level, Gleason score, and clinical stage, and models risk on a continuous scale, rather than classifying patients into discrete risk groups. Because risk groups can often be heterogeneous, outcome predictions can be less accurate than continuous models. External validation of the nomogram demonstrated a concordance index of 0.61 to 0.64. Calibration of the nomogram indicated that the actual outcome probabilities of this tool may be as much as 5% better or 30% worse than that predicted by the nomogram. The nomogram is shown in Fig. 2.

In a recent analysis of the Memorial Sloan-Kettering Cancer Center experience using intraoperative conformal treatment planning for permanent implan-

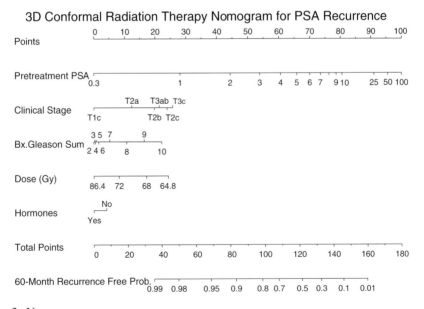

FIG. 2. Nomogram

tation, the biochemical outcomes for favorable-risk patients were compared with those for similar patients treated with intensity-modulated radiotherapy (IMRT) to dose levels of 81 Gy. With a median follow-up of three years in each group, the biochemical outcomes for the brachytherapy group and the high-dose IMRT group were 95% and 93%, respectively (unpublished data). D'Amico et al. [19] recently compared the outcome for low-risk patients treated between 1997 and 2002 with radical prostatectomy ($n = 322$) and MRI-guided I-125 implantation ($n = 196$). With a median follow-up of four years, the five-year PSA control rates for patients treated with surgery and brachytherapy were 93% and 95%, respectively.

Sequelae of LDR Brachytherapy; Acute and Late Toxicity

Transient urinary morbidity related to radiation-induced urethritis or prostatitis represents the most common side effect after prostate brachytherapy. The symptoms include urinary frequency, urinary urgency, and dysuria. Because of the varying definitions of toxicity reported in the literature, it is difficult to quantify the true risks of treatment-related toxicities after seed implantation. Many reports have not described toxicity outcomes using actuarial methods, and in some studies only severe toxicity is reported while more moderate complications (grade 2) are not reported. In addition, various implantation techniques, seed activity, and source distribution patterns used by different centers have contributed to the wide range of side-effect profiles reported after prostate brachytherapy.

Acute Urinary Retention

Acute urinary retention (AUR) is a known risk that can occur immediately after prostate brachytherapy. Locke et al. [20] reported the experience from Seattle in 62 consecutive patients followed after prostate brachytherapy. In that prospective study, all patients were evaluated with baseline AUA scores, urodynamic assessments, and prostate-volume assessments. The patients were contacted at monthly intervals to obtain accurate follow-up information. Catheterization was required in 42% (26 of 62) of the patients. The incidence of urinary retention was 34% at one week, 29% at one month, and 18% at three months from completion of the procedure. Among many variables analyzed, a prostate volume $>33\,cm^3$ was an independent predictor of AUR. Other reports in the literature have indicated much lower incidences of AUR after prostate brachytherapy. Crook et al. [21] studied 150 patients treated with prostate brachytherapy between 1999 and 2001. In this group, 13% ($n = 20$) developed AUR. Of these 20 patients, 55% received neoadjuvant androgen deprivation (NAAD) therapy to decrease the size of the prostate prior to the procedure. A multivariate analysis revealed that larger prostate volumes and prior hormone therapy were each independent predictors of AUR.

Terk et al. [22] reported on 251 patients treated with TPI; 137 patients were implanted with I-125 and 114 were treated with Pd-103. Overall, urinary retention requiring catheterization in more than 48 h developed in 5.5% of patients. Among patients with preimplantation International Prostate Symptom Score (IPSS) >20, 10–20, and <10, the rates of acute urinary retention after TPI were 29%, 11%, and 2%, respectively. One recent report [23] demonstrated an association between the volume of the transitional zone (TZ) noted on MRI and the incidence of AUR. Among patients with MRI-defined TZ volumes of <50, 50–60, and >60 cm³, the incidence of AUR was 0% (0/40), 33% (1/3), and 71% (5/7), respectively. In a multivariate analysis, Crook et al. [24] observed that only the baseline urinary function and the IPSS score were predictors of AUR, whereas the TZ index was not a significant predictor of this endpoint. These data, in combination with the lack of correlation of AUR with the dose delivered to the urethra or prostate, suggest that the etiology of AUR is most likely related to trauma to the prostate gland.

Urinary Tolerance

In general, almost all patients after prostate brachytherapy develop acute urinary symptoms such as urinary frequency, urinary urgency, and occasional urge incontinence. Depending upon the isotope used, these symptoms often peak at one to three months after the procedure and subsequently gradually decline over the ensuing three to six months. Most patients significantly benefit from the use of an alpha-blocker, which ameliorates such symptoms in 60% to 70% of patients.

Grimm et al. [25] summarized the tolerance outcome in 310 patients who received I-125 or Pd-103 for localized disease. During the first 12 months after the procedure, approximately 90% of the patients had grade 1 or 2 acute urinary symptoms, which included urinary frequency, urinary urgency, and obstructive symptoms. Grade 3 acute toxicity was reported in 8% of patients, and 1.5% experienced a grade 4 toxicity. Late grade 3 and 4 toxicities were noted in 7% and 1%, respectively. These authors also documented urinary incontinence rates ranging from 6% to 48% among patients with a prior history of TURP. Among those patients without a history of TURP and with modest gland volumes, the incidence of chronic urethritis and incontinence was found to be less than 3%.

The five-year tolerance outcome of CT-preplanned implantation at Memorial Sloan-Kettering Cancer Center was reported by Zelefsky et al. [26]. One hundred thirty-five patients (55%) developed acute grade 2 urinary symptoms after permanent I-125 interstitial implantation. These symptoms included urinary frequency and urgency, which were generally treated with alpha-blocker medications. Patients were characterized as having late grade 2 urinary toxicity if acute symptoms persisted for more than one year after TPI or had become clinically manifest at that time. One hundred patients (40%) developed late grade 2 urinary toxicity, and the five-year actuarial likelihood of grade 2 urinary toxicity was 41%. These symptoms often persisted in these patients during the first year after seed implantation and were effectively managed with alpha-blocker therapy. The actuarial likelihood of grade 2 urinary symptom resolution at one, two, and three years after TPI was 19%, 50%, and 70%, respectively. Twenty-three patients (9%) developed urethral strictures after brachytherapy (grade 3 urinary toxicity). The five-year likelihood of stricture development was 10%, and the median time to development was 18 months.

Brown et al. [27] reported on 87 patients who underwent prostate brachytherapy and whose urinary symptoms were carefully assessed after the procedure. Urinary effects such as frequency, nocturia, and dysuria generally developed two to three weeks postimplantation and peaked three to four months after the procedure. A gradual decline in the severity of symptoms was noted in approximately 75% of the patients during the first 12 months. In this series, 41% of the patients experienced acute grade 2 or 3 urinary morbidity, with 6% having acute grade 3 urinary morbidity. After 12 months, 22% of the patients experienced persistent urinary morbidity. Of this latter group, approximately 70% were characterized as having persistent grade 1 and 30% as having persistent grade 2 or 3 symptoms.

According to the aforementioned reports, there appears to be a higher incidence of acute grade 2 genitourinary symptoms with standard implantation techniques than with conformal radiotherapy. The increased likelihood of such symptoms is related to the higher doses inevitably delivered to the urethra, which generally average 1.5 to 2 times more than the prescription dose. The uniform source and needle placement initially used by the Seattle group were associated with central doses that were in excess of 200% of the prescription dose. These observations influenced these investigators to use a modified peripheral seed-loading approach to minimize the urethral dose to 150% or less of the prescription dose. Several reports have noted that acute urinary symptoms and late urinary morbidity after seed implantation correlate with the central target doses and the proximity of seed placement to the urethra. Others [28] demonstrated a reduction in grade 2 symptoms (from 42% to 19%) when the central dose was reduced by placement of half-strength radioactive seeds in the periurethral area. Wallner et al. [29] demonstrated a correlation of late urethral toxicity with the urethral dose from prostate brachytherapy. In that study, the average maximal urethral dose among patients with late grade 2 and 3 urinary toxicities was 592 Gy, compared with 447 Gy for those who had minimal (grade 1) or no late urinary toxicity ($p = 0.03$).

With the introduction of intraoperative conformal planning for ultrasound-based implantation at Memorial Sloan-Kettering Cancer Center in 1996, a significant reduction in the average and maximal urethral doses achieved with this approach translated into an improved urinary tolerance profile and quality of life for treated patients. Zelefsky et al. [30] reported a reduced incidence of grade 2 acute urinary symptoms and more rapid resolution of symptomatology with this technique compared with a preplanned technique previously used at the institution (Fig. 3). These data highlight the important relationship between the urethral dose and urinary symptoms after prostate brachytherapy. Careful

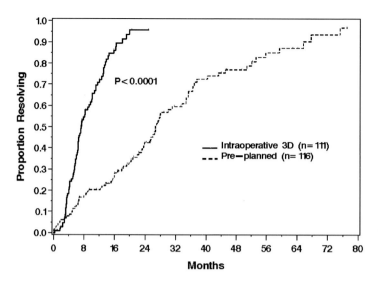

Fig. 3. Time to urinary symptom resolution

attention to this parameter during intraoperative planning is important for achieving an optimal outcome, and a modified peripherally loaded implant not in conjunction with computer-generated planning will not necessarily consistently achieve lower urethral doses.

Rectal Tolerance

The reported incidence of grade 2 rectal toxicity after prostate brachytherapy ranges from 2% to 12%. Grade 3 or 4 rectal toxicity is unusual (<2%). Grimm et al. [25] reported grade 2 late proctitis in 2% to 12% of patients treated at the Seattle Prostate Institute, but no grade 3 or 4 gastrointestinal complications were reported. The actuarial incidence of late grade 2 rectal bleeding was 9%. In general, such symptoms were treated with conservative measures and resolved in all cases. One patient (0.4%) developed a grade 4 rectal complication.

Waterman and Dicker [31] reported on the dosimetric predictors of late rectal toxicity in 98 patients who were treated with I-125 implantation. Based on dose-surface histograms performed in all cases, late rectal morbidity correlated strongly with the percentage of the rectal surface that received at least 100 Gy. The probability of late rectal morbidity was 0.4%, 1.2%, and 4.7% when the maximal rectal dose was 150, 200, and 300 Gy, respectively. According to that report, constraining the rectal dose to 100, 150, and 200 Gy to 30%, 20%, and 10% of the rectal surface, respectively, should result in less than 5% rectal morbidity. Snyder et al. [32] also observed a correlation between the volume of the rectum irradiated to the prescription dose and late rectal toxicity after prostate brachytherapy. The five-year likelihood of rectal toxicity was 18% for patients in whom more than 1.3 cm³ of rectal tissue was exposed to 160 Gy or higher, compared with a 5% incidence among patients in whom less than 1.3 cm³ of the rectum was exposed to these dose levels. The incidence of rectal toxicity correlated with the volume irradiated: 0% for 0.8 cm³, 7% to 8% for >0.8 to 1.8 cm³, and 25% for >1.8 cm³. Meticulous attention to needle and seed placement in the operating room as well as intraoperative dose-volume histograms of normal tissue should reduce the rectal doses and the risks of toxicity to minimal levels.

Erectile Function

Although reports have noted relatively low rates of impotence after prostate implantation [33], this endpoint was only evaluated at two years after implantation. There is a paucity of long-term data critically examining this issue. Stock et al. [33] also reported gradually declining erectile function with continued follow-up after brachytherapy in 89 patients. However, the median follow-up in that report was only 15 months. It appears that impotence rates after TPI are probably underestimated in the literature. With longer follow-up observations, Zelefsky et al. [3] reported that whereas the incidence of impotence two years after implantation was 21%, the rate increased to 42% five years after the procedure.

Although the development of erectile dysfunction after prostate brachytherapy is likely to be a multifactorial phenomenon, the influence of the dose of radiation to the penile bulb may be an important variable. Merrick et al. reported a 61% six-year actuarial rate of erectile dysfunction [34]. Factors that predicted an increased risk of posttreatment impotence included the preimplantation potency score, the use of supplemental external-beam radiotherapy, and diabetes. These authors also reported an association between higher doses to the penile bulb and the development of impotence after seed implantation [35]. In that report, among 75% of the men who developed erectile dysfunction, the dose to 50% of the penile bulb exceeded 40% of the prescription dose. On the other hand, among 90% of the patients who remained potent after therapy, the dose to 50% of the penile bulb was estimated to be less than 40% of the prescription dose. In a multivariate analysis, the following parameters were significant predictors of erectile dysfunction after brachytherapy: the D50 to the penile bulb, the postimplantation prostate CT volume, and the patient's age. Yet one should note that these investigators typically place a significant percentage of seeds in extraprostatic regions, which may have contributed to these findings. Kitely et al. [36] could not establish this association, yet in their report, the implant technique used at their institution did not require the placement of the radioisotope outside of the prostatic capsule.

Improved erectile function has been observed after sildenafil citrate use in the treatment of impotence after brachytherapy. In one report, 80% of patients responded well to the medication [37]. These results are consistent with similar responses reported with this medication for prostate cancer patients with erectile dysfunction after external-beam radiotherapy [38]. In one study [39], the addition of neoadjuvant androgen deprivation had a significant impact on the potency preservation rate after prostate brachytherapy. Among patients treated with brachytherapy alone who developed impotence after implantation, 30 of 37 (81%) responded to sildenafil, as compared with a response rate of 22 of 48 (46%) for patients who received neoadjuvant androgen deprivation therapy in combination with brachytherapy ($p = 0.04$).

Future Directions in Prostate Brachytherapy: Integrating Biologic-Based Imaging Information into Treatment Planning

Reports from investigators at the University of California San Francisco have indicated that magnetic resonance spectroscopy (MRS) may provide reliable information regarding the ability to more precisely localize malignant zones within the prostate gland [40]. MRS takes advantage of the significantly higher choline levels and significantly lower citrate levels in regions of cancer compared to regions of benign prostatic hypertrophy and normal prostatic epithelium. Detection was especially enhanced when magnetic resonance imaging was combined with MRS, with specificity and sensitivity of detection of abnormal zones within the prostate as high as 91% and 95%, respectively. While it is well recognized that prostate cancers are often multifocal, MRS may provide valuable information to highlight regions in the prostate that contain the most densely populated zones of biologically active disease. This information could then be used to design more optimal radiotherapy treatment plans and facilitate dose escalation.

A potential advantage of incorporating MRS data into brachytherapy treatment-planning algorithms is the ability to escalate radiation doses to intraprostatic regions that correspond to positive voxels noted on the MRS. Dose escalation with permanent interstitial brachytherapy may potentially have the most impact for improving outcome among patients with intermediate-risk prognostic features. Although dose escalation may be unnecessary among patients with favorable-risk prostate cancer using transperineal brachytherapy, the outcome for patients with intermediate prognostic features may be improved with the delivery of higher doses. Inferior outcomes with brachytherapy alone for intermediate or unfavorable risk disease could possibly be related to the inability of intraprostatic implanted seeds to adequately treat the periprostatic tissue, which is likely to contain microscopic disease extension. Alternatively, such patients may have tumors with a higher volume of radioresistant clones and may require higher intraprostatic radiation doses to effectively eradicate disease.

We have previously demonstrated the feasibility of integrating the information from MRI and spectroscopy into intraoperative treatment plans with the intention of selectively escalating the dose to abnormal regions to 150% of the prescription dose levels [41]. More recently, we updated our experience with

MRSI-guided dose escalation in 44 patients with clinically localized prostate cancer (unpublished data). The ratios of choline and citrate for the prostate were analyzed, and regions of high risk for malignant cells were identified. The co-ordinates of abnormal voxels identified on MRS were transferred and overlaid on the intraoperative ultrasound images. A computer-based intraoperative con-formal treatment-planning system was used to determine the optimal seed dis-tribution to deliver a prescription dose of 144 Gy to the target volume (prostate), 200% to 300% of the prescription dose to the abnormal regions identified on MRS, and to maintain the urethral and rectal doses within tolerance ranges. The MRSI-identified abnormal voxels received a mean dose of 343 Gy (238% of the 144 Gy prescription dose). The minimum dose delivered to the MRS-abnormal voxels was 182 Gy (126% of the prescribed target dose). Despite the dose esca-lation achieved for the MRS-positive voxels, the urethral and rectal doses were maintained within tolerance ranges. The median average rectal and urethral doses were 49% and 130% of the prescription dose. The percentages of patients with acute grade 2 gastrointestinal toxicity 6 and 12 months after implantation were both 2%. The percentages of patients with acute grade 2 genitourinary tox-icity 6 and 12 months after implantation were 30% and 14%, respectively. The percentage of patients with late grade 2 gastrointestinal toxicity 12 months after implantation was 7%. The percentage of patients with late grade 2 genitourinary toxicity 12 months after implantation was 18%. One patient (2%) developed late grade 3 genitourinary toxicity (urethral stricture), and no patients developed late grade 3 or higher gastrointestinal toxicity.

Further studies will be necessary to fully explore the specificity and sensitiv-ity of MRS and its pathologic correlation with radical prostatectomy specimens. These data, nevertheless, indicate that new biologic-based imaging modalities may have profound implications for improving the targeting ability of radio-therapeutic interventions. Such approaches will probably allow escalated radia-tion doses to be delivered to limited regions within the target volume that harbor the greatest concentration of tumor clonogens without exceeding normal tissue tolerance levels and hence improve the therapeutic ratio.

References

1. Bealieu L, Aubin S, Taschereau R, Poiliot J, Vigneault E (2002) Dosimetric impact of the variation of the prostate volume and shape between pre-treatment planning and treatment procedure. Int J Radiat Oncol Biol Phys 53:215–221
2. Stone NN, Roy J, Hong S, et al (2002) Prostate gland motion and deformation caused by needle placement during brachytherapy. Brachytherapy 1:154–160
3. Zelefsky MJ, Yamada Y, Cohen G, et al (2000) Postimplantation dosimetric analysis of permanent transperineal prostate implantation: improved dose distributions with an intraoperative computer-optimized conformal planning technique. Int J Radiat Oncol Biol Phys 48:601–608
4. Yu Y, Zhang JBY, Brasacchio RA, et al (1999) Automated treatment planning engine for prostate seed implant brachytherapy. Int J Radiat Oncol Biol Phys 43:647–652

5. Lee EK, Gallagher RJ, Silvern D, et al (1999) Treatment planning for brachytherapy: an integer programming model, two computational approaches and experiments with permanent prostate implant planning. Phys Med Biol 44:145–165

6. Wilkinson DA, Lee EJ, Ciezki JP, et al (2000) Dosimetric comparison of pre-planned and OR-planned prostate seed brachytherapy. Int J Radiat Oncol Biol Phys 48:1241–1244

7. Matzkin H, Kaver I, Bramante-Schreiber L, et al (2003) Comparison between two iodine-125 brachytherapy implant techniques: pre-planning and intra-operative by various dosimetry quality indicators. Radiother Oncol 68:289–294

8. Nguyen J, Wallner K, Han B, Sutlief S (2002) Urinary morbidity in brachytherapy patients with median lobe hyperplasia. Brachytherapy 1:42–47

9. Zelefsky MJ, Whitmore WF, Leibel SA, et al (1993) Impact of transurethral resection on the long-term outcome of patients with prostatic carcinoma. J Urol 150:1860–1864

10. Blasko JC, Ragde H, Grimm PD (1991) Transperineal ultrasound-guided implantation of the prostate: morbidity and complications. Scand J Urol Nephrol 137:113–117

11. Wallner K, Lee H, Wasserman S, et al (1997) Low risk of urinary incontinence following prostate brachytherapy in patients with a prior transurethral prostate resection. Int J Radiat Oncol Biol Phys 37:565–569

12. Stone NN, Ratnow ER, et al (2000) Prior transurethral resection does not increase morbidity following real time ultrasound-guided prostate seed implantation. Tech Urol 6:123–127

13. Grann A, Wallner K (1998) Prostate brachytherapy in patients with inflammatory bowel disease. Int J Radiat Oncol Biol Phys 40:135–138

14. Grimm PD, Blasko JC, Sylvester JE, Meier RM, Cavanagh W (2001) 10-year biochemical (prostate-specific antigen) control of prostate cancer with I-125 brachytherapy. Int J Radiat Oncol Biol Phys 51:31–41

15. Blasko JC, Grimm PD, Sylvester JE, et al (2000) Palladium 103 brachytherapy for prostate carcinoma. Int J Radiat Oncol Biol Phys 46:839–850

16. Prestidge BR, Hoak DC, Grimm PD, et al (1997) Posttreatment biopsy results following interstitial brachytherapy in early stage prostate cancer. Int J Radiat Oncol Biol Phys 37: 31–39

17. Kollmeier MA, Stock RG, Stone N (2003) Biochemical outcomes after prostate brachytherapy with 5-year minimal follow-up: importance of patient selection and implant quality. Int J Radiat Oncol Biol Phys 57:645–653

18. Kattan MW, Potters L, Blasko JC, et al (2001) Pretreatment nomogram for predicting freedom from recurrence after permanent prostate brachytherapy in prostate cancer. Urology 58:393–399

19. D'Amico AV, Tempany CM, Schultz D, et al (2003) Comparing PSA outcome after radical prostatectomy or magnetic resonance imaging-guided partial prostatic irradiation in select patients with clinically localized adenocarcinoma of the prostate. Urology 62:1062–1067

20. Locke J, Eliis W, Wallner K, Cavanagh W, Blasko J (2002) Risk factors for acute urinary retention requiring temporary intermittent catheterization after prostate brachytherapy: a prospective study. Int J Radiat Oncol Biol Phys 52:712–719

21. Crook J, McLean M, Catton C, et al (2002) Factors influencing risk of acute urinary retention after TRUS-guided permanent prostate seed implantation. Int J Radiat Oncol Biol Phys 52:453–460

22. Terk MD, Stock RG, Stone NN (1998) Identification of patients at increased risk for prolonged urinary retention following radioactive seed implantation of the prostate. J Urol 160:1379–1382

23. Merrick GS, Butler WM, Galbreath RW, et al (2001) Relationships between the transition zone index of the prostate gland and urinary morbidity after brachytherapy. Urology 57:524–529

24. Crook J, Toi A, McLean M, Pond G (2002) The utility of transition zone index in predicting acute urinary morbidity after 125-I prostate brachytherapy. Brachytherapy 1:131–137

25. Grimm PD, Blasko JC, Ragde H, et al (1996) Does brachytherapy have a role in the treatment of prostate cancer? Hematol Oncol Clin North Am 10:653–673

26. Zelefsky MJ, Hollister T, Raben A, et al (2000) Five year biochemical outcome and toxicity with transperineal CT-planned permanent I-125 prostate implantation for patients with localized prostate cancer. Int J Radiat Oncol Biol Phys 47:1261–1266

27. Brown D, Colonias A, Miller R, et al (2000) Urinary morbidity with a modified peripheral loading technique of transperineal (125) I prostate implantation. Int J Radiat Oncol Biol Phys 47:353–360

28. Stokes SH, Real JD, Adams PW, et al (1997) Transperineal ultrasound-guided radioactive seed implantation for organ confined carcinoma of the prostate. Int J Radiat Oncol Biol Phys 37:337–341

29. Wallner KE, Roy J, Harrison L, et al (1995) Dosimetry guidelines to minimize urethral and rectal morbidity following transperineal I-125 prostate brachytherapy. Int J Radiat Oncol Biol Phys 32:465–471

29. Stock RG, Stone NN, Lo YC (2000) Intraoperative dosimetric representation of the real-time ultrasound implant. Tech Urol 6:95–98

30. Zelefsky MJ, Yamada Y, Marion C, et al (2003) Improved conformality and decreased toxicity with intraoperative computer-optimized transperineal ultrasound-guided prostate brachytherapy. Int J Radiat Oncol Biol Phys 55:956–963

31. Waterman FW, Dicker AP (2003) Probability of late rectal morbidity in 125-I prostate brachytherapy. Int J Radiat Oncol Biol Phys 55:342–353

32. Snyder KM, Stock RG, Hong SM, Lo YC, Stone NN (2001) Defining the risk of developing grade 2 proctitis following I-125 prostate brachytherapy using a rectal dose volume histogram analysis. Int J Radiat Oncol Biol Phys 50:335–341

33. Stock RG, Stone NN, Iannuzzi C (1996) Sexual potency following interactive ultrasound-guided brachytherapy for prostate cancer. Int J Radiat Oncol Biol Phys 35:267–272

34. Merrick GS, Butler WM, Galbreath RW, et al (2002) Erectile function after permanent prostate brachytherapy. Int J Radiat Oncol Biol Phys 52:893–902

35. Merick GS, Butler WM, Wallner KE, et al (2002) The importance of radiation doses to the penile bulb vs. crura in the development of postbrachytherapy erectile dysfunction. Int J Radiat Oncol Biol Phys 54:1055–1062

36. Kitely RA, Lee WR, deGuzman AF, et al (2002) Radiation dose to the neurovascular bundles or penile bulb does not predict erectile dysfunction after prostate brachytherapy. Brachytherapy 1:90–94

37. Merrick GS, Butler WM, Lief JH, et al (1999) Efficacy of sildenafil citrate in prostate brachytherapy patients with erectile dysfunction. Urology 53:1112–1116

38. Zelefsky MJ, McKee AB, Lee H, et al (1999) Efficacy of oral sildenafil in patients with erectile dysfunction after radiotherapy for carcinoma of the prostate. Urology 53:775–778

39. Potters L, Torre T, Fearn PA, et al (2001) Potency after permanent prostate brachytherapy for localized prostate cancer. Int J Radiat Oncol Biol Phys 50:1235–1242
40. Yu KK, Scheidler J, Hricak H, et al (1999) Prostate cancer: prediction of extracapsular extension with endorectal MR imaging and three-dimensional proton MR spectroscopic imaging. Radiology 213:481–488
41. Zelefsky MJ, Cohen G, Zakian KL, et al (2000) Intraoperative conformal optimization for transperineal prostate implantation using magnetic resonance spectroscopic imaging. Cancer J 6:249–255

Targeting Energy-Assisted Gene Delivery in Urooncology

Yasutomo Nasu, Fernando Abarzua, and Hiromi Kumon

Summary. Applications of energy sources which were applied for endourology is discussed with special reference to efficient targeting gene delivery for the treatment of urological cancer. Gene therapy has attracted attention as a possible solution to many major diseases, such as cancer and cardiovascular disorders. The urogenital organs are excellent specific targets for the application and evaluation of gene therapy. Most gene therapy strategies have already been applied to urological cancers, with an acceptable safety profile but with limited clinical benefits and many hurdles to overcome. The efficient and safe delivery of therapeutic genes in vivo remains a major challenge to the realization of gene-based therapeutic strategies. Local injection of therapeutic gene (in situ gene therapy) is currently practical way with maximum efficacy and safety. Shock waves and ultrasound, therapeutic energies which were developed for endourology, have the potential to enhance the transfection efficiencies in a variety targeted tissues and cell types. Targeting energy-assisted local gene delivery into urologic organs using endourological techniques can be possible and will be one of the most effective modalities in the future endourooncology.

Keywords. Gene therapy, Shock wave, Ultrasound, HIFU, endourooncology

Research on therapeutic applications of various energy sources has created innovative and effective treatment tools in the field of urology. In this decade, various techniques, such as radiofrequency therapy (see the chapter by S. Kanazawa, this volume), cryosurgery (see the chapter by K. Nakagawa, this volume), interstitial thermotherapy, brachytherapy (see the chapter by M. Zelefsky, this volume), and high-intensity focused ultrasound (see the chapter by T. Uchida, this volume) have been introduced as minimally invasive treatments in endourology. Recent advances in these fields have been discussed intensively in this book. In this chapter, new application of energy sources which were applied for endourology is discussed, with special reference to efficient targeting gene delivery.

Department of Urology, Okayama University Graduate School of Medicine and Dentistry, 2-5-1 Shikata, Okayama 700-8558, Japan

Gene Therapy in Urology

There are many situations in medicine and biology in which it is desired to introduce a macromolecule into the cytoplasm of mammalian cells. One important application is gene therapy, where it is necessary to deliver a gene or a synthetic oligonucleotide into a cell. Gene therapy has attracted attention as a possible solution to many major diseases, such as cancer and cardiovascular disorders [1].

Current gene therapy is regarded as translational research from the bench to the bedside, which must go back to the bench after the clinical data have been obtained. The urogenital organs are excellent specific targets for the application and evaluation of gene therapy. Since conventional cytokine therapy and adoptive immunotherapy are clearly effective against renal-cell carcinoma, it is appropriate to incorporate them in immune gene therapy using cytokine gene transfer and tumor-cell vaccination. Bladder tumors have shown excellent response to intravesically administered immune response modifiers, such as interferon and bacillus Calmette-Guérin. Intravesical administration is a simple and reliable way of delivering the genetic agent, and cystoscopy and urinary cytology will be helpful in evaluating the response of the tumor to treatment. For prostate cancer, direct intratumoral injection under ultrasonographic guidance is also a simple and effective way to deliver the genetic agent, and prostate-specific antigen (PSA) is an extremely sensitive marker for therapeutic effectiveness.

Basic strategies for clinical gene therapy that have been studied include immune gene therapy using cytokine gene transfer and tumor-cell vaccination, gene replacement therapy using tumor suppressor genes, antisense therapy inhibiting activated oncogenes, and "suicide gene" therapy activating selective prodrugs [2]. All four of these strategies have already been applied to urological cancers, presenting an acceptable safety profile but with limited clinical benefits and many hurdles to overcome [3]. At this time point, local and direct injection of the therapeutic gene into a targeted organ or lesion, in situ gene therapy, is the most practical way of clinical gene therapy with maximum efficacy and safety. The efficient and safe delivery of therapeutic genes in vivo remains a major challenge to the realization of gene-based therapeutic strategies.

Gene Delivery and Energy Sources

Increasing attention has been paid to technology used for the delivery of genetic materials into cells for gene therapy and the generation of genetically engineered cells. So far, viral vectors have been mainly used because of their inherently high gene transfection efficiency [3]. However, there are some problems to be resolved for clinical applications, such as the pathogenicity and immunogenicity of the viral vectors themselves. Therefore, many research trials with nonviral vectors have been performed to improve their efficiency to a level comparable to that of the viral vector. These research trials have developed in two directions: material improvement of nonviral vectors and their combination with various external physical stimuli.

Plasma membranes consist of lipid bilayers that are highly impermeable to DNA and other negatively charged macromolecules, leading to the search for methods of temporarily increasing membrane permeability without consequent cytotoxicity. A range of methods to achieve this goal has been reported, including microinjection [4], biolistics (high-velocity particles or gene gun) [5], electroporation [6], chemical methods [7], shock waves [8], and ultrasound [9]. Although these methods have demonstrated an enhancement of transfection efficiencies in a variety of tissues and cell types, widespread clinical application of many gene transfer strategies awaits further improvements in gene transfer methodology and elucidation of the mechanism.

Shock wave and ultrasound, therapeutic energies which were developed for endourology, have been studied extensively in vitro and in vivo among those strategic methods. Merging of endourological techniques and gene therapeutic techniques have the possibility to enhance and facilitate the development of the treatment for urologic malignancies. In situ cancer gene therapy based on endourological techniques will be one of the powerful modality in future. Detail and future aspects are discussed.

Shock Waves

Background

Shock-wave lithotripsy is widely used for treatment of urolithiasis. Research into broader application of this energy source has shown some promise in the treatment of malignant tumors. As a direct action, shock waves can induce mechanical damage in tumor cells via acoustic cavitation [10, 11]. Shock waves can also facilitate the transfer of large molecules into cells, which provides an explanation for the findings that combined therapy overcomes the resistance of some tumors to chemotherapy alone. Combination treatments with shock waves and biological response modifiers [12] or chemotherapy [13] have shown enhancement of the therapeutic results for some tumors.

In Vitro

Cell permeabilization using shock waves is a way of introducing macromolecules and small polar molecules into the cytoplasm [14]. Shock waves can deliver molecules up to a molecular weight of 2,000,000 into the cytoplasm of cells without toxicity [15]. Transmembrane molecular delivery depends on the shock-wave pressure profile and impulse of the shock waves (pressure integrated over time). Shock waves also change the permeability of the nuclear membrane and transfer molecules directly into the nucleus.

The transfer of molecules into cells by shock waves can include even such large molecules as DNA plasmids capable of subsequently expressing marker proteins, and therapeutic proteins, which directly suggested the possibility of human gene therapy by shock-wave treatment. Schaaf et al. [16] showed that naked plasmid

DNA can easily and effectively be delivered to malignant urothelial cells in vitro upon exposure to lithotripter-generated shock waves.

In Vivo

The potential for gene transfection during shock-wave tumor therapy in vivo was evaluated by searching for shock-wave-induced DNA transfer in B16 mouse melanoma tumor cells [17]. A luciferase reporter vector and air at 10% of tumor volume were injected before shock-wave exposure to promote cavitation. Shock-wave exposure enhanced luciferase expression in cells isolated immediately after treatment, and also in cells isolated after 1 day, which demonstrated gene expression within the growing tumors. With the use of the same treatment methods with a reporter plasmid coding for green fluorescent protein (GFP) [18], 2 days after exposure to 400 shock waves, the recovery of viable cells from excised tumors was reduced to 4.2% of shams, and cell transfection was enhanced, reaching 2.5% of cell counts ($p < 0.005$, t-test). These results show that tumor ablation induced by shock-wave treatment can be coupled with simultaneous enhancement of gene transfection, which supports the concept that gene and shock-wave therapy might be advantageously merged.

In vivo treatment experiments were conducted using a therapeutic gene and its recombinant protein [19]. The effects of shock waves, recombinant interleukin-12 (rIL-12) protein, and DNA plasmids coding for interleukin-12 (pIL-12) on the progression of mouse B16 melanoma and RENCA renal carcinoma tumors were investigated. Shock-wave treatment consisted of 500 shock waves (7.4 MPa peak negative pressure) from a spark-gap lithotripter. The combination of shock waves and pIL-12 injection produced a statistically significant reduction in tumor growth relative to shock waves alone for both tumor models. IL-12 expression due to shock-wave-induced gene transfer was confirmed in ELISA assays. This research demonstrates a potentiality for further development of shock-wave-enhanced cancer gene therapy. Nasu et al. investigated the efficacy of a single injection of a recombinant adenovirus expressing murine IL-12 (AdmIL-12) directly into orthotopic mouse prostate carcinomas [20]. Significant growth suppression and suppression of pre-established lung metastases were observed following the injection of AdmIL-12 into the orthotopic tumor. Based on this preclinical study, a clinical trial for prostate cancer was initiated using a recombinant adenovirus expressing human IL-12. The combination of IL-12 gene therapy (direct injection of adenovirus vector expressing IL-12 into prostate) and shock-wave treatment for prostate cancer may be possible in the future.

Future Directions

Shock-wave-enhanced cancer gene therapy has biphasic effects, with direct cell killing due to cavitation and cell killing caused by gene transduction. The relative proportion of these effects depends on the condition of the shock waves applied. The effect of the cavitation bubbles created by lithotripter-generated shock waves is also implicated in the mechanism of lithotripter-induced cell and tissue damage. When the pressure waves propagate in human tissues, side effects such as vascular damage and hematoma are induced. It must be ensured that the shock-wave parameters needed for effective cell permeability do not cause unacceptable tissue damage in vivo. Further studies will be necessary to understand the mechanism of shock-wave-induced uptake of molecules, focusing on the shock-wave impulse, the subsequent shear force against the cells, the change in membrane permeability of different cell types, and ionic charge.

Ultrasound

Ultrasound is best known for its imaging capability in diagnostic medicine. However, there have been considerable efforts recently to develop therapeutic uses for ultrasound [21]. Ultrasound has been utilized to enhance the delivery and effect of three distinct therapeutic drug classes: chemotherapeutic, thrombolytic, and gene-based drugs. In addition, ultrasound contrast agents have recently been developed for diagnostic ultrasound. New experimental evidence suggests that these contrast agents can be used as exogenous cavitation nuclei for enhancement of drug and gene delivery. In comparison with diagnostic ultrasound, progress in the therapeutic use of ultrasound has been somewhat limited. Recent successes in ultrasound-related drug-delivery research have positioned ultrasound as a therapeutic tool for drug delivery in the future. Recent advances in these fields are discussed below.

Ultrasound-Mediated Gene Delivery

The use of ultrasound in therapeutic medicine is a developing field. The effects of ultrasound have been evaluated in terms of the biological changes induced in the structure and function of tissues [22]. The main fields of study have been in sonodynamic therapy, improving chemotherapy, gene therapy, and apoptosis therapy. The expression level of plasmid DNA by various cationized polymers and liposomes is promoted by ultrasound irradiation in vitro as well as in vivo [23]. Ultrasound irradiation under appropriate conditions enables cells to accelerate the permeation of the cationized gelatin-plasmid DNA complex through the cell membrane, resulting in enhanced transfection efficiency of plasmid DNA. These findings clearly indicate that ultrasound exposure is a simple and promising method to enhance the gene expression of plasmid DNA (Fig. 1) [24].

These experiments were performed using nonfocused low-pressure ultrasound waves, in contrast to the focused ultrasound discussed later.

Ultrasound Contrast Agent and Gene Delivery

Transfection with ultrasound and microbubbles has been reported as a powerful new tool in gene therapy. New experimental evidence suggests that these contrast agents can be used as exogenous cavitation nuclei for enhancement of drug and gene delivery [25].

170   Y. Nasu et al.

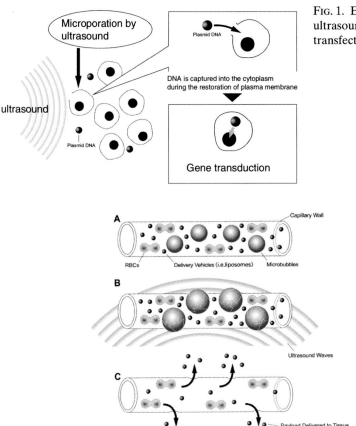

Fig. 1. Enhancement of ultrasound-mediated gene transfection

Fig. 2. Schematic representation of a method for delivering intravascular drugs or genes to tissues with microbubbles. **A** Intravascular microbubbles and gene-bearing vehicles flow through capillaries. **B** Ultrasound is applied in the target region, thereby destroying the microbubbles and permeabilizing the microvessel wall. **C** Intravascular gene-bearing vehicles are delivered to the tissue by convective forces. *RBCs*, Red blood cells

Ultrasound contrast agent microbubbles, which are typically used for image enhancement, are capable of amplifying both the targeting and the transport of drugs and genes to tissues. Microbubble targeting can be achieved by the intrinsic binding properties of the microbubble shells or through the attachment of site-specific ligands. Once microbubbles have been targeted to the region of interest, microvessel walls can be permeabilized by destroying the microbubbles with low-frequency, high-power ultrasound (Fig. 2).

A second level of targeting specificity can be achieved by carefully controlling the ultrasound field and limiting microbubble destruction to the region of interest. When microbubbles are destroyed, drugs or genes that are housed within them or bound to their shells can be released to the blood stream and then deliv-

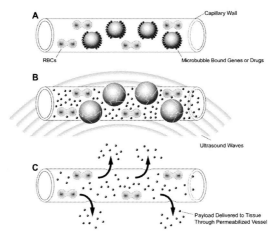

Fig. 3. Schematic representation of a method for delivering intravascular drugs or genes to tissues with microbubbles that are engineered to house drugs or genes on the microbubbles. **A** Intravascular microbubble-bound genes or drugs flow through capillaries. **B** Ultrasound application to the target region destroys microbubbles, thereby permeabilizing the microvessel walls and releasing drugs or genes into the blood stream. **C** Drugs or genes are delivered to tissue through permeabilized microvessels by convective forces

ered to tissue by convective forces through the permeabilized microvessels. An alternative strategy is to increase the payload volume by coinjecting drug- or gene-bearing vehicles, such as liposomes, with the microbubbles. In this manifestation, microbubbles are used for creating sites of microvessel permeabilization that facilitate drug or gene vehicle transport (Fig. 3) [25]. Azuma et al. established a novel ultrasound contrast agent-mediated gene transfection approach and demonstrated the significant prolongation of graft survival by the successful transfection of NFkappa B-decoy into the donor kidney in a rat renal allograft model [26].

The major problem with these methods is the relatively low efficiency of the gene transfer ratio compared with other methods, such as the use of virus vectors, particularly in vivo. Further, the amount of contrast agent necessary to obtain satisfactory transduction efficiency is significantly higher than that recommended for clinical use. Modification of the plasma membrane on which transient pore formation occurs influences the transduction efficiency. Local anesthetics as membrane modifiers were shown to enhance the efficiency of ultrasound-mediated gene transfection with an echo contrast agent. Local anesthetics have been shown to destabilize lipid membranes by breaking the hydration shell and fluidizing lipid membranes [27]. This enhancement effect by local anesthetics could be useful for ultrasound-mediated gene therapy in the future, since both methods of membrane modification could be directly applied to the human body.

HIFU for gene tranduction

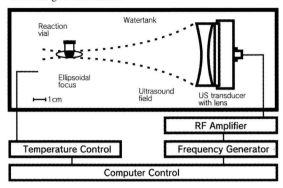

FIG. 4. Schematic representation of high-intensity focused ultrasound (HIFU) device. Focused ultrasound was generated by a piezoelectric disc transducer, focused by a polystyrene lens, and coupled into a water tank. The reaction vials containing cells mixed with DNA were positioned in the ellipsoidal focus. For in vivo experiments, the same device was used

HIFU (High-Intensity Focused Ultrasound) and Gene Delivery

High-intensity focused ultrasound (HIFU) is a noninvasive surgical technique in which ultrasound energy is delivered transcutaneously to a discrete area within the body. The efficacy of HIFU has been demonstrated in the treatment of prostatic disease [28]. Preliminary experience with the use of HIFU in the treatment of renal-cell carcinoma has been reported [29, 30].

HIFU also has the potential to assist in the noninvasive spatial regulation of gene transfer into the targeted tissue [31]. In contrast with low-pressure ultrasound, HIFU waves can be focused on different anatomical locations in the human body, including the prostate, kidney, and bladder, without significant adverse effects.

Huber et al. showed that HIFU can significantly enhance the transfection of plasmid DNA in the Dunning prostate tumor R3327-AT1 in vitro and in vivo after direct plasmid injection without marked side effects (Fig. 4) [32]. This enhancement could be demonstrated by means of histological analysis, as well as by quantitation of gene expression using ELISA assay. It was also indicated that ultrasound interaction mechanisms other than heat are probably responsible for transfection enhancement. Nevertheless, focused ultrasound-induced gene transfection could be favorably combined with the thermal effects of focused ultrasound occurring at increasing intensities, especially in cancer therapy. Noninvasive HIFU therapy, in combination with ultrasound-induced transfer of drug-activating genes such as cytosine diaminase or the herpes simplex thymidine kinase genes, could result in an interesting and realistic locoregional tumor treatment option.

Further analysis for mechanism, safety evaluation, and determination of ideal treatment conditions will be necessary for actual clinical application. In this research, experience and data obtained in endourological practice using various energy sources are useful. Concordant development of basic gene therapy research and endourology will make a great contribution to the innovation of new treatment methods especially for urologic cancer. For the future development of endourooncology, merging of endourological techniques and gene therapeutic techniques is one of the direction to pursue as a translational research.

References

1. Kumon H (2000) Status and prospects of gene therapy for urologic cancer. Mol Urol 4:39–40
2. Nasu Y, Kusaka N, Saika T, Tsushima T, Kumon H (2000) Suicide gene therapy for urogenital cancer: current outcome and prospects. Mol Urol 4:67–71
3. Nasu Y, Djavan B, Marberger M, Kumon H (1999) Prostate cancer gene therapy: outcome of basic research and clinical trials. Tech Urol 5:185–190
4. Davis BR, Yannariello-Brown J, Prokopishyn NL, Luo Z, Smith MR, Wang J, Carsrud ND, Brown DB (2000) Glass needle-mediated microinjection of macromolecules and transgenes into primary human blood stem/progenitor cells. Blood 95:437–444
5. Furth PA (1997) Gene transfer by biolistic process. Mol Biotechnol 7:139–143
6. Ho SY, Mittal GS (1996) Electroporation of cell membranes: a review. Crit Rev Biotechnol 16:349–362
7. Spiller DG, Giles RV, Grzybowski J, Tidd DM, Clark RE (1998) Improving the intracellular delivery and molecular efficacy of antisense oligonucleotides in chronic myeloid leukemia cells: a comparison of streptolysin-O permeabilization, electroporation, and lipophilic conjugation. Blood 91:4738–4746
8. Mulholland SE, Lee S, McAuliffe DJ, Doukas AG (1999) Cell loading with laser-generated stress waves: the role of the stress gradient. Pharm Res 16:514–518
9. Gambihler S, Delius M, Ellwart JW (1994) Permeabilization of the plasma membrane of L1210 mouse leukemia cells using lithotripter shock waves. J Membr Biol 141:267–275
10. Delius M (1994) Medical application and bioeffects of extracorporeal shock waves. Shock Waves 4:55–72
11. Gamarra F, Spelsberg F, Dellian M, Goetz AE (1993) Complete local tumor remission after therapy with extra-corporeally applied high-energy shock waves (HESW). Int J Cancer 19;55:153–156
12. Oosterhof GO, Smits GA, de Ruyter AE, Schalken JA, Debruyne FM (1991) Effects of high-energy shock waves combined with biological response modifiers in different human kidney cancer xenografts. Ultrasound Med Biol 17:391–399
13. Weiss N, Delius M, Gambihler S, Eichholtz-Wirth H, Dirschedl P, Brendel W (1994) Effect of shock waves and cisplatin on cisplatin-sensitive and -resistant rodent tumors in vivo. Int J Cancer 58:693–699
14. Kodama T, Hamblin MR, Doukas AG (2000) Cytoplasmic molecular delivery with shock waves: importance of impulse. Biophys J 79:1821–1832
15. Kodama T, Doukas AG, Hamblin MR (2002) Shock wave-mediated molecular delivery into cells. Biochim Biophys Acta Jan 30;1542:186–194

16. Schaaf A, Langbein S, Knoll T, Alken P, Michel MS (2003) In vitro transfection of human bladder cancer cells by acoustic energy. Anticancer Res 23:4871–4875

17. Bao S, Thrall BD, Gies RA, Miller DL (1998) In vivo transfection of melanoma cells by lithotripter shock waves. Cancer Res 58:219–221

18. Miller DL, Bao S, Gies RA, Thrall BD (1999) Ultrasonic enhancement of gene transfection in murine melanoma tumors. Ultrasound Med Biol 25:1425–1430

19. Song J, Tata D, Li L, Taylor J, Bao S, Miller DL (2002) Combined shock-wave and immunogene therapy of mouse melanoma and renal carcinoma tumors. Ultrasound Med Biol 28:957–964

20. Nasu Y, Bangma CH, Hull GW, Lee HM, Hu J, Wang J, McCurdy MA, Shimura S, Yang G, Timme TL, Thompson TC (1999) Adenovirus-mediated interleukin-12 gene therapy for prostate cancer: suppression of orthotopic tumor growth and pre-established lung metastases in an orthotopic model. Gene Ther 6:338–349

21. Ng KY, Liu Y (2002) Therapeutic ultrasound: its application in drug delivery. Med Res Rev 22:204–223

22. Yu T, Wang Z, Mason TJ (2004) A review of research into the uses of low level ultrasound in cancer therapy. Ultrason Sonochem 11:95–103

23. Hosseinkhani H, Aoyama T, Ogawa O, Tabata Y (2003) Ultrasound enhances the transfection of plasmid DNA by non-viral vectors. Curr Pharm Biotechnol 4:109–122

24. Hosseinkhani H, Aoyama T, Ogawa O, Tabata Y (2002) Ultrasound enhancement of in vitro transfection of plasmid DNA by a cationized gelatin. J Drug Target 10:193–204

25. Price RJ, Kaul S (2002) Contrast ultrasound targeted drug and gene delivery: an update on a new therapeutic modality. J Cardiovasc Pharmacol Ther 7:171–180

26. Azuma H, Tomita N, Kaneda Y, Koike H, Ogihara T, Katsuoka Y, Morishita R (2003) Transfection of NFkappaB-decoy oligodeoxynucleotides using efficient ultrasound-mediated gene transfer into donor kidneys prolonged survival of rat renal allografts. Gene Ther 10:415–425

27. Nozaki T, Ogawa R, Feril LB Jr, Kagiya G, Fuse H, Kondo T (2003) Enhancement of ultrasound-mediated gene transfection by membrane modification. J Gene Med 5:1046–1055

28. Mulligan ED, Lynch TH, Mulvin D, Greene D, Smith JM, Fitzpatrick JM (1997) High-intensity focused ultrasound in the treatment of benign prostatic hyperplasia. Br J Urol 79:177–180

29. Kohrmann S, Kohrmann KU, Michel MS, Gaa J, Marlinghaus E, Alken P (2002) High intensity focused ultrasound as noninvasive therapy for multilocal renal cell carcinoma: case study and review of the literature. J Urol 167:2397–2403

30. Wu T (2003) Preliminary experience using high intensity focused ultrasound for the treatment of patients with advanced stage renal malignancy. J Urol 170:2237–2240

31. Huber PE, Mann MJ, Melo LG, Ehsan A, Kong D, Zhang L, Rezvani M, Peschke P, Jolesz F, Dzau VJ, Hynynen K (2003) Focused ultrasound (HIFU) induces localized enhancement of reporter gene expression in rabbit carotid artery. Gene Ther 10:1600–1607

32. Huber PE, Pfisterer P (2000) In vitro and in vivo transfection of plasmid DNA in the Dunning prostate tumor R3327-AT1 is enhanced by focused ultrasound. Gene Ther 7:1516–1525

Subject Index